MEDICAL ASTROLOGY

Let the Stars Guide You to Good Health

DIANE CRAMER, M.S.

JOVE
PRESS

Printed in the U.S.A.
ISBN 978-0-9821691-1-7

Jove Press
420 E. 80th Street, Suite 10G
New York City, NY 10075
www.bobmarksastrologer.com

Acknowledgements

I want to thank Bob Marks for his help and support over the years and for making the publication of this book possible. Also thanks to my sister, Ronnie Cramer, for her valuable insight and advice. Thanks also to Terry Marks for her superb design and formatting of the book and her infinite patience with the numerous editing changes.

Disclaimer

The material in this book is for instructional purposes only and is not intended, nor meant to replace or to be used for the purpose of a medical diagnosis or treatment. Ms. Cramer is not a medical doctor nor physician. For a medical diagnosis – see a licensed medical doctor or physician.

INTRODUCTION

In the following pages you will be introduced to the many facets of medical astrology. You will gain an understanding of how the planets, signs and aspects work in medical astrology. You will learn how to identify strengths and weaknesses in the natal chart as well as proneness to specific disorders. Predictive techniques are included to help you identify times of stress. Valuable information on astrology and nutrition is included as well as special techniques to help you fine tune your medical astrology expertise.

The contents of this book are taken from a variety of lectures given over the years by Diane Cramer at several NCGR conferences in New York City. Though the lectures have been edited to make them more readable, in most cases they are still in lecture format and in many cases include audience questions and answers. In some cases additional information has been added to the original lecture. A brief description of each lecture is included preceding each chapter. The variety of topics will appeal to both beginners and advanced students of astrology. There are several case studies and examples to illustrate various techniques in medical astrology. Specific diseases and health issues are studied.

KEY OF SYMBOLS

♈	Aries	☉	Sun
♉	Taurus	☽	Moon
♊	Gemini	☿	Mercury
♋	Cancer	♀	Venus
♌	Leo	♂	Mars
♍	Virgo	♃	Jupiter
♎	Libra	♄	Saturn
♏	Scorpio	♅	Uranus
♐	Sagittarius	♆	Neptune
♑	Capricorn	♇	Pluto
♒	Aquarius	ASC	Ascendant
♓	Pisces	MC	Midheaven
'	Minutes of Arc	℞	Retrograde
⚶	Vesta	☌	Conjunction
⚳	Ceres	✳	Sextile
⚷	Chiron	□	Square
⚵	Juno	△	Trine
⚴	Pallas-Athena	⚻	Quincunx
☊	Moon's North Node	☍	Oppostion

CONTENTS

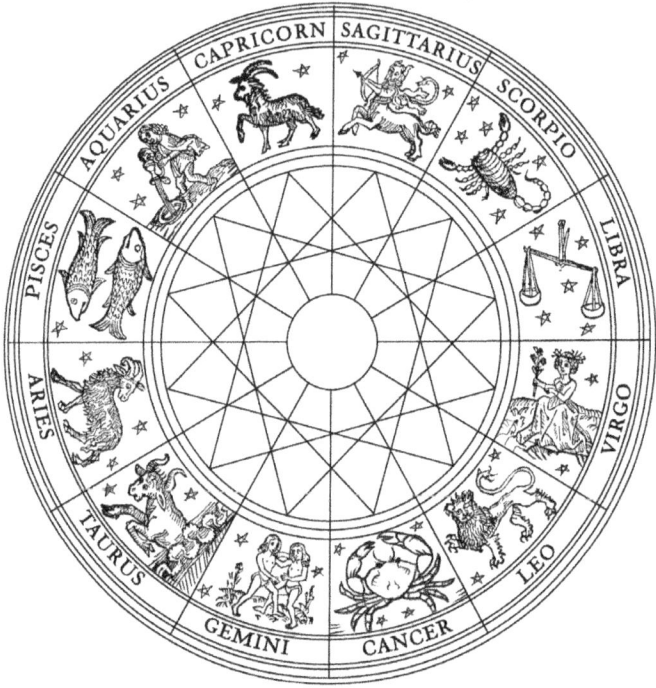

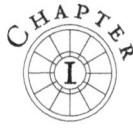

THE PLANETS
IN MEDICAL ASTROLOGY

An understanding of the planets in medical astrology is essential to evaluating a chart in terms of health. The following chapter includes the meanings of the planets in both the natal chart and in predictive use as well as planetary combinations and midpoints.

This chapter will describe how the planets interact with each other in terms of medical astrology. We aren't forgetting the signs and houses, but the focus is on the planets. I always like to mention that no matter what you see in a chart – you can see some very difficult combinations or you can see combinations that aren't so difficult – it doesn't necessarily mean something is going to happen to you in terms of health. It also doesn't mean that if you think you have a good chart then you will never be ill. One must always be diligent in regards to their own health.

You also can't ignore heredity; you have to consider age and how well you take care of yourself when evaluating a chart. If you know anything about health and you study health, then you can solve some of your problems especially if you know what it means when you have certain aspects in your chart. What am I lacking based on the aspects? What do I need to build up in my body? When you get into medical astrology you will learn how to evaluate health in a chart.

I'm going to start with the planets individually. Then we'll look at them in midpoint combination, then in prediction. We'll do aspects. And we'll go through some charts and try to understand particular health issues.

The planets in the chart interact with each other and can point to various health disorders and the nature of the planets affect the severity of illness. I wanted to mention a book that I've just rediscovered that I've had for many years. This is an old medical astrology book called *Medical Astrology*[1] by Henreich Daath that was first reprinted in 1968. It doesn't include Pluto and for a long time I didn't understand the concepts in the book, but I looked at it again recently and realized it really does explain the actions of the planets in medical astrology in terms of a planet working positively, a planet's energies suppressed, a planet working unnaturally or perverted in relation to illness. I highly recommend this book even though it doesn't cover Pluto as it was originally written before Pluto was discovered or at least understood by astrologers.

THE SUN ☉

The Sun is really one of the two luminaries. In terms of the planets in medical astrology, if you have difficult aspects involving your Sun, you can have an energy problem. There can be a problem in keeping your vitality at an even level, but it can also indicate low ego energy. An afflicted Sun can result in inflammation or infection. And you start with the Sun, as it's the most obvious. And when you're checking a chart you can see how well you withstand disease, how you fight against disease, or your vitality based on the aspects to the Sun and midpoint combinations involving the Sun. Generally, the Sun has to do with your energy and vitality and if it is afflicted – let's say it's hit by a difficult transit – you could have a fever or inflammation.

THE MOON ☽

The Moon has rulership over the fluids in our bodies. The Moon can refer to emotional issues, but it also has to do with women's cycles and diurnal cycles. It is involved with fluid retention, discharges, mucous, water retention – all these have to do with the Moon. Secretions in the body, tears, anything that is watery is associated with the Moon.

When the Sun and Moon are in hard aspect you can have vitality problems. Or you can have eye problems. It's one of the significators of problems with the eyes and, of course, there are other significators.

MERCURY ☿

Mercury has to do with respiratory problems and also rules the nervous system. I also think it is involved with the hormones of the body because Mercury is the messenger planet. I believe Pluto has to do with the endocrine system as a whole and Mercury rules the action of the hormones. That is because hormones are chemical messengers in the body. But with Mercury respiratory problems can also show up.

I wanted to explain what I meant when I say you're getting a particular problem involving a planet. Let's assume a planet is afflicting your Mercury. You might be subject to asthma, bronchitis, that sort of thing. However, it's never just one significator in the chart. There are usually several significators that could lead to a disease. So when I'm giving a health reading, and I see someone has three or four significators pointing to a particular problem, I consider the situation borderline. When I see someone has several afflictions that all lead to the same thing – for example the throat or respiratory system, I tell them it's much more difficult in the chart and shows a proneness to a specific type of illness. So I've learned over the years to see what's borderline, such as a mildly afflicted Mercury, you might have weak nerves, for example. If you see several indications of a condition, and it will include houses and angles – Mercury on an angle, for example, receiving many hard aspects – that will be much more difficult than Mercury in a cadent house getting maybe one difficult aspect as far as the severity of your problem. The planets show duration of disease which I will discuss in transits and progressions while the severity of the problem is based on how afflicted the planet is in the chart and how much is going on at one time in your chart. And I think in medical astrology all the old rules on good and bad aspects work.

So Mercury is also the nervous system. When I see the charts of people who have a lot of afflictions with Mercury or involving the mutable cross, since Mercury rules two signs in the mutable cross – Gemini and Virgo, then they may experience nervous disorders. That's one of the meanings of afflictions involving Mercury or the mutable cross. The main issues can be respiratory and can also involve the nervous system. Also a hormonal imbalance can show up as a Mercury problem.

VENUS ♀

Now, what is Venus in medical astrology? Venus rules sweets so it has to do with insulin. Venus is the venous circulation; Jupiter is the arterial circulation of the body. Venus is sugar; Jupiter is fat. So problems with the liver and fat assimilation are a Jupiter problem. Problems with sugar metabolism are a Venus problem. I like to think of conditions in terms of pairs as it helps you to see the difference between the two.

Blood sugar problems would include an afflicted Venus. And phlebitis would be a Venus problem – an afflicted Venus in the chart because it rules the veins, but arteriolosclerosis involves the arteries which is a Jupiter problem. Do you see the difference? Venus is also involved in the equilibrium of the body and body chemistry.

Both Venus and Jupiter could have to do with blood including also Mars in that Mars rules the red blood cells. Venus is a benign growth. Usually it's something simple that can be easily removed. Venus also shows up in a transit as a lack of tone in the body. You're just out of shape with Venus. Basically Venus rules sugar and carbohydrates.

MARS ♂

When we get to Mars we start to get real afflictions because with Mars you've got inflammation; you've got bruising. It rules surgery, wounds, blood ailments and fevers. Pluto can be a higher octave of Mars so where Mars can be an infection that you get over in a few days Pluto can be a massive infection. If you have Mars and Pluto in aspect in your chart, you may be prone to long-term infections. That's how you try to learn medical astrology – by combining the planets. Inflammation is Mars, and you should be aware that Mars rules acidity, acids. Think of it in contrast to Saturn, which is alkaline. So you've got your acid-alkaline imbalance showing with your Mars and Saturn. (Acid-alkaline imbalance can also be seen in an afflicted Venus. See Chapter Seven for more information on acid-alkaline imbalance.) Now if your chart has a strong Mars, then you're more subject to inflammation.

If you chart has a stronger Saturn than Mars, then you may be more prone to stiffness. This is another method. You try to contrast the planets in your chart. William Davidson whose medical astrology book[2] of his lectures was published in 1979 did a lot of this contrasting, and he always said to see which planet is stronger in your chart – what you're prone to. So see what is stronger in your chart. Saturnine problems if Saturn is strong in your chart are stiffness, alkalinity and hardening. If you're more Martian, you going to experience inflammatory or infectious type of problems, also bruising. And Mars afflictions can also indicate surgery as well as a sexual dysfunction.

Mars rules the red blood cells so when there's an affliction with Mars it can sometimes indicate anemia. It also can be that your adrenals are not working up to par. You're not fighting off disease well. You can build up your adrenals; you can build up the weak parts of the body. So Mars is fevers. If you combine the Sun and Mars you can get a high fever as they both have to do with feverish types of complaints.

JUPITER ♃

Jupiter, as mentioned rules fats, also the liver function in the body. Jupiter can also be swelling in the body. Diseases caused by excess such as gout are a Jupiterian type of problem. Jupiter rules the arterial blood and conditions such as arteriolosclerosis. I have seen many heart problems in the chart show up with a Jupiter Saturn combination. So there's something about Jupiter Saturn in aspect, Saturn restricting the blood flow or causing clotting or some other problem to indicate heart disease. (See Chapter Three for a more complete discussion of heart disease).

SATURN ♄

Saturn is associated with the bones; it rules the teeth. It's any structural problem in the body which is why it shows up as arthritis and rheumatism; also dental problems, problems with hearing – deafness. It will probably not work alone; it can be in aspect to Mercury if you are going to have a problem with hearing, but it's still going to be an afflicter in that way. Chronic disease is Saturnine; acute disease is Martian. So if it's quick and you get over it fast, it's Mars. If you hold onto it a long time, it's Saturn. Under activity is Saturn. The sign ruling the part of your body that Saturn tenants is the weakest part of the body. It gets the least blood supply. Therefore, it's the weakest organ in your body and needs to be nourished. The sign position of Neptune is similar to Saturn, but there's a flabbiness with Neptune. Sometimes flabbiness has to do with Neptune and Venus combinations also.

Audience: Can you please repeat what you just said about Saturn.

DC: Those organs related to the sign tenanted by Saturn are considered to be the weakest parts of the body. So if you have Saturn in Taurus the throat area can be weak.

Then I said that the sign placement of Neptune is similar to Saturn, but it is not so much weak as flabby. It has a lack of tone. The organ in your body ruled by the sign Neptune resides in needs to be built up.

Now many more people were born with Neptune in the same sign than Saturn, so it's more generational than Saturn. Neptune still seems to point out a weak area, and there is less blood going to the organ ruled by Saturn's sign placement. Calcifying and hardening – these are all Saturn issues too.

URANUS ♅

Now Uranus has to do with conditions of spasm or seizure, anything sudden or unusual. Unusual is Neptune also. The very unusual or weird diseases are Uranian or Neptunian. Something twisted in your body is Uranus. Cramps. Electrical shocks – anything like that has to do with the planet Uranus. So it would show up with epilepsy, for example. But I doubt it would work alone. Epilepsy would also involve Mercury. Assimilation of oxygen in the body can be Uranus also.

NEPTUNE ♆

In medical astrology, there's no getting around it. Neptune is the culprit. It really is the problem planet as far as I'm concerned in medical astrology. It's the most difficult. It can be diseases that show up without advance warning, like a cancer throughout your body. With other planets such as Saturn, you start to see a problem beforehand such as a tumor and you can work on getting rid of it. With Neptune it's much more difficult.

Let's look at Jackie Kennedy Onassis's chart. She had Neptune conjunct the MC. There's an elevated Neptune in a critical degree conjunct the MC. I know there are a few charts going around for her, but I've seen this one enough times that I believe it's the correct chart. 00 degrees and 29 degrees are critical degrees. So obviously that's going to make a situation worse or more intense. So she has a 00 degree Neptune conjunct the MC of almost 29 degrees and Neptune rules the immune system. And she had Non-Hodgkin's lymphoma. And she didn't live a long time after it was diagnosed. Looking at her chart, I didn't find a lot of obvious problems. I just wanted to use this chart to point out an example of how Neptune can be a very difficult, insidious planet.

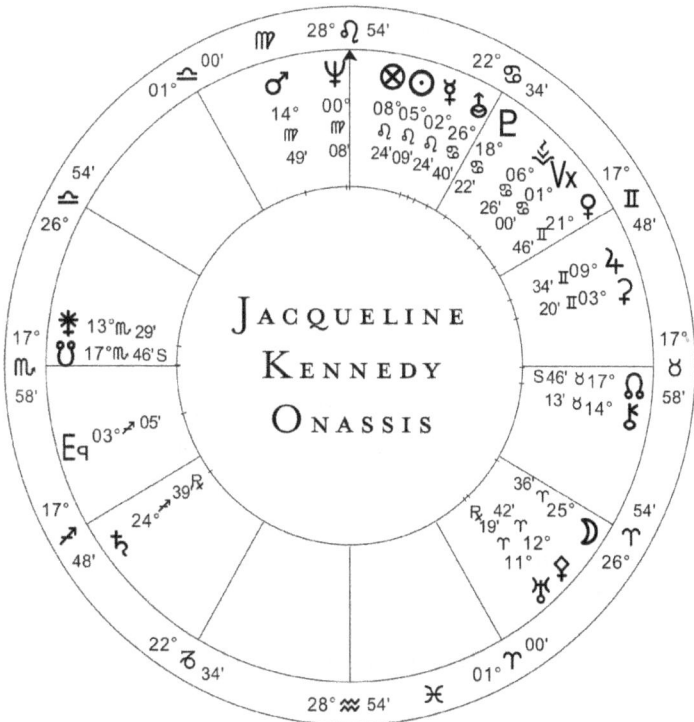

JACQUELINE KENNEDY ONASSIS

Neptune is also misdiagnosis, hidden illness and also rules a coma though usually it's a Moon Neptune combination for a coma. And of course drug addition, alcoholism and poisoning are associated with Neptune. If you have an afflicted Neptune in your chart, I would advise you to get one of those books on building up your immune system. It's a difficult planet. Neptune in combination with the Sun can be a vitality problem.

PLUTO ♇

Now, in terms of Pluto it may have something to do with hereditary diseases when it shows up on an angle. There are other indictors that show up as hereditary, but I think Pluto is one indication. It also rules birth defects, malformation and amputation. By the way, just take this information as information on a planet. Otherwise medical astrology can upset some people. Operations, and as I said before, massive infection are ruled by Pluto. Mars can be infection, but Pluto can be massive infection. Both can be involved with surgery. Anything drastic is Pluto, like a transplant. I would expect to see a strong Plutonian influence for a transplant.

Those are the basic meanings of the planets in medical astrology. I should also mention Pluto has to do with the endocrine system as I said earlier, the reproductive system and regeneration. A badly aspected Pluto can mean that you have to go through a crisis and then you regenerate, and you're in better shape for it. It is not necessarily something the opposite.

Audience: What about the common cold?

DC: I would say it's a Mercury problem. If you get a lot of colds, possibly you have a poorly aspected Mercury, as Mercury rules respiratory illness. I found that when I started taking vitamin and mineral supplements, I went from six colds a year to no colds in ten years. And I also changed the way I ate. That's why I believe in nutrition. And it's how I got into medical astrology because the day I started studying astrology I also began studying nutrition. It was in the 1980's that I saw a book on medical astrology and realized that was what I was meant to do – learn medical astrology.

Another thing we should look at, going back to Jackie Kennedy Onassis's chart, notice Mars is in her 10th house with Neptune. Most of the difficult problems with the immune system, and it could be colds, are Mars Neptune – a very difficult combination. And it shows up as a lowered immune function, with cancer, AIDS, etc. Also Mars in Pisces can be difficult. So if you have a difficult aspect in your chart between Mars and Neptune you really should get on any kind of program that enhances the immune system. There are many books on enhancing your immune system.

Audience: Didn't you say something about Neptune having something to do with allergies?

DC: Yes, but usually the Moon is also involved. There's something about the Moon and Neptune, angular, elevated, or in the sixth house that has to do with allergies. Mercury is associated with allergies too. Again that's respiratory allergies. If you have stomach allergies, the Moon will be involved. And Saturn and Venus would be involved with skin allergies.

You have to learn your rulerships. I'm giving you a lot of information, but it's only a small portion of what you need to know in medical astrology. And I always like to add – never use medical astrology to diagnose. Even a doctor who is also a medical astrologer would not use medical astrology to diagnose. Use it to confirm. See how long you might have a condition. See what you're prone to. See your strengths and weaknesses. Never diagnose with medical astrology. Because you can't. For example, a hard aspect between Jupiter and Saturn could be anything from the liver to the gallbladder to hardening of the arteries. How do you know which one it is? You might find out by using the signs and the houses, but you should never diagnose with medical astrology. There are too many variables. And you have to be a doctor to diagnose illness.

Audience: What about the fifth house as an indication of the Sun?

DC: I would check the fifth house in terms of heart disease to see if there were malefic planets along with an afflicted Sun.

Audience: But in terms of being indicative of something since the Sun rules the fifth house.

DC: It doesn't work that way.

Audience: But the aspects? I'm asking you because in one week thousands and thousands of people are born with the same aspects all over the world. That means they are not all going to have the same thing. And the houses are more personal.

DC: Right. The time of birth makes the chart more personal and focuses the energy in various parts of the chart. Aspects to the angles are used in determining proneness to disease. There are cardinal, fixed and mutable types of diseases. And you have to determine what you're prone to. Does that make sense? (This idea is expanded on throughout this book.) You can definitely take a chart, just like you do with your love life and your personality and get a variety of information. It doesn't matter when they were born. It all depends on the rising sign and what's hitting the angles.

Let's go to midpoints. And then we'll discuss planetary combinations and predictions.

MIDPOINTS

It was in Marcia Starck's first book on medical astrology where I first read about the six major medical midpoints.[3] I find they work. You look to see what is hitting these midpoints: the Sun/Moon midpoint, the Mars/Saturn midpoint, the Mars/Uranus midpoint, the Mars/Neptune midpoint, the Mars/Pluto midpoint, and the Saturn/Neptune midpoint.

Again, I have seen the charts of people with very good aspects to the Sun/Moon midpoint, and they contracted a disease so I decided that during their lives they are living well. There are other indications in the chart as to why something happens to you.

So you can look to see if something equals your Sun/Moon midpoint. Obviously, if Saturn or Neptune equals your Sun Moon midpoint, your vitality can be low or there is the potential for illness.

Mars/Saturn. If a planet equals Mars/Saturn that organ does not develop well, or there can be illness in that part of the body. It is also involved in bone inflammation. Mars/Uranus midpoint combinations show up in those who have surgery. A planet or an angle equals the Mars/Uranus midpoint such as MC = Mars/Uranus; Sun = Mars/Uranus. It's definitely a surgery aspect. Also, cuts, nervous disorders, injuries, accidents.

Now Mars/Neptune is toxicity. Also poisoning, drugs. It's also another allergy significator. It's another combination to consider besides the Moon and Neptune for allergies and also for examining the immune function. For example, let's look at Robert Urich's chart. He first developed cancer in 1996. His MC and Moon; if you look at his chart, he's got the Moon in 20° Scorpio 31" and the 1C is 19° Scorpio 56" both equal by conjunction to Mars/Neptune. The Mars/Neptune midpoint is 21° Scorpio 19". And Moon/MC = Mars/Neptune by square – very, very strong. I have found that indirect midpoints work too. This happens to be a direct midpoint – Moon = Mars/Neptune; MC = Mars/Neptune.

Do you understand the difference between a direct and an indirect midpoint? The direct midpoints are the conjunction and opposition and the indirect are the square, sesquiquadrate and semisquare. I find they all work. Some say only the conjunction and the opposition are strong, but that's not necessarily so. This is an example of Mars/Neptune toxicity hitting two personal points in the chart by direct midpoint. And he got cancer. Mars/Neptune brings in the susceptibility for infection. So that's where the body is weak. Now Scorpio rules the colon in the chart, so there is a weakness there and it needs to be built up. Now it's very simplistic, but I'm just giving you an

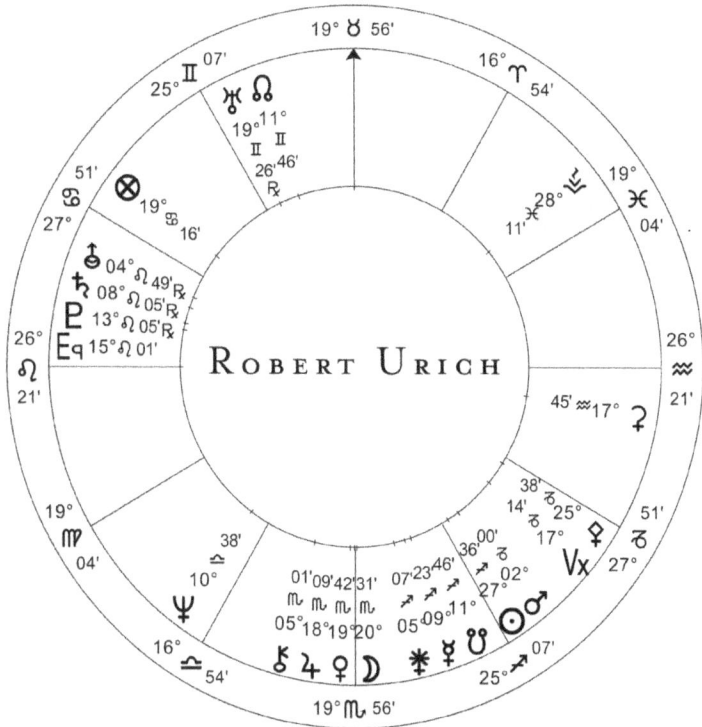

ROBERT URICH

example of what you can do to try to solve a problem. If we think of Mars/Neptune as the immune function of the body, then there's a problem. Because two personal points equal that midpoint.

AUDIENCE: How do you know what part of the body is affected?

DC: Look at the sign of the midpoint; in this case it was in Scorpio. Of course you should go farther and look at the whole fixed cross. And then say to yourself, "This part of my body may be subject to infection or may be weak. I'd better work on it."

If this were a woman's chart, you might think your reproductive area could be weak too. It doesn't mean that women don't get colon problems because Audrey Hepburn died of colon cancer. So though there are men's and women's diseases, it's also a part of the body that could be weak. And, of course, using polarities the other side could be weak too – the throat – Taurus or the thyroid. And of course in a male chart Scorpio can also refer to the prostate.

You have to be aware of your signs. But in this chapter I'm focusing on the planets.

Where a planet falls at the midpoint, you look at the sign and see if you can build up that part of the body.

The Mars/Pluto midpoint has to do with the endocrine system, the colon, destruction of cells and heavy accidents. Just the two in aspect is not a great combination. Mars/Saturn and Saturn/Neptune are difficult in terms of health. They are involved in the structures of the body. There can be a weakness at the point of Saturn/Neptune. Everybody does not have a planet falling at one of these points. I print out the midpoint trees, and I look to see. Sometimes somebody might have a planet at one of these points; sometimes not. You just check the chart. And you look for a whole lot of indicators to check the severity of a problem. And some astrologers will do transits to the midpoints. This brings in more information or confirmation of a health issue.

Saturn/Neptune is a weak point in the body just like Mars/Saturn. I find them similar. There's something not right at that point in the body. It can mean a disease at that point or a slowly developing illness.

Here are some midpoint combinations that refer to bodily weakness.

Neptune = Mars/Saturn
Ascendant = Moon/Neptune
Neptune = Moon/Uranus
Jupiter = Sun/Neptune
Sun = Mars/Neptune or Saturn = Mars/Neptune
Ascendant = Mars/Neptune.

Another useful midpoint is Mars/Jupiter: It is involved in reproduction issues, fertility and the timing of childbirth.

The following is the chart of a stroke victim.

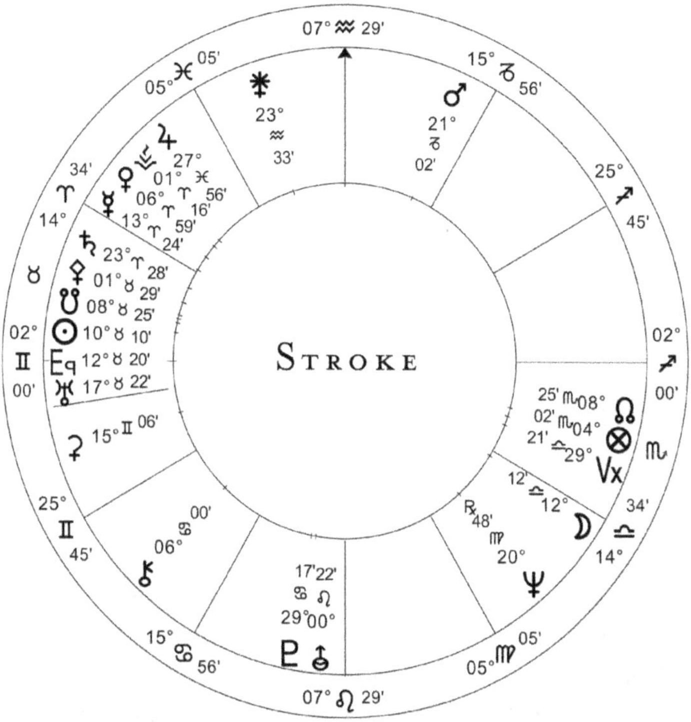

AUDIENCE: How old was she when she had the stroke?

DC: She was in her early 50's. What I thought was interesting was that there is a hard aspect between Mercury and Mars which is not that strong but Mercury and Mars can refer to the way you use your hands, and she can't use one of her hands very well since the stroke. And interesting, Mercury/Mars equals her Ascendant. There's also Saturn in Aries because all those planets in Aries can have to do with a problem with the head or a stroke. The Venus in Aries equals Mars/Neptune and Saturn/Neptune. So I just felt those midpoints harmed this area – the head area (Aries) and she did have a stroke. And there's a Mars square Saturn aspect also. That can also be a health problem.

AUDIENCE: She has Mars trine Neptune.

DC: That may be why she is ok. She has mostly recovered. The worst that happened is that after she recovered she had limited use of one of her hands, but other wise she's fine.

AUDIENCE: The Mercury conjuncts Venus.

DC: Yes, it's all pulled in. Notice that she has all those planets in the 12th house. She works in a hospital.

Let's look at another chart with an example of a Mars Neptune aspect. Look at the first breast cancer chart. What do you see rising and elevated in the chart – Mars and Neptune. This is a person who took good care of herself. She didn't eat junk food, but she has this aspect. There's something wasting about Mars and Neptune together. I have a chart of a man who has Lou Gehrig's disease (See

Chapter Two) and the Mars and Neptune are in mundane square – the wasting away of muscles can be Mars and Neptune. Now this wasn't a muscle case. Mars rules the muscles and with Mars Neptune in hard aspect, it can be some kind of wasting disease. In this case it's a problem with the immune system with Mars Neptune. By the way, she was a very talented artist. And that's another emphasis that I find in the charts of artists – a strong Neptunian aspect – and that's why they are so creative or they get an immune disorder disease, or they become alcoholics or drug addicts.

BREAST CANCER

AUDIENCE: Might that Mars work in terms of the house it rules as well?

DC: It can have an influence over the house it rules, but as far as the rules of medical astrology, it's an angular situation with an elevated planet. And that makes it strong. There's also Mars quincunx Saturn. And Neptune is square the Ascendant. What's giving her strength? The Sun is trine Saturn. She tried to cure herself with natural ways. She didn't want surgery. However, the natural ways did not work. She since had a mastectomy, chemotherapy and almost died of a brain tumor, started to recover, then eventually passed on. And as awful as these stories are of chemotherapy and radiation, the natural methods didn't do anything to help her. She only got worse. And this is a person who all her life was into natural ways and ended up getting cancer. And she couldn't figure that out. And then she tried to cure it naturally, but it doesn't work. I think there's something about endurance and structure when Saturn makes a good aspect to the Sun. The Sun trine Saturn may have helped for awhile. She also had the Sun opposite Pluto. And that can be a degenerative aspect. She managed to finish some difficult art work before she died even though she didn't have a lot of energy. That's an example of the aspects in action.

AUDIENCE: I wonder if you use the chart ruler or the ruler of the Ascendant as I noticed in the breast cancer chart before that Saturn is the ruler of the chart conjunct Uranus but it's sextile Pluto and that seems like something favorable in the long run.

DC: The ruler of the Ascendant is very important especially if it's being hit by transit in terms of duration of a health disorder. Whenever I give a general reading, I don't usually get a lot into health issues. The most I'll describe are periods of high and low vitality or stress or tell someone to use caution as you're more prone to infection; be careful of eating in restaurants or being around large crowds. I'll mention infection if I see someone is going to have a difficult Neptune transit. Be careful of food poisoning. I might tell somebody that. You don't want to lay a trip on someone and create a lot of anxiety in their life.

AUDIENCE: She also has Moon opposite Saturn that is not so good.

DC: Well, as I mentioned she eventually passed on so the good aspects kept her going for a while but eventually nothing helped.

Audience: There's one other thing. Mercury rules her sixth house which is treatment. And it's in Capricorn which is traditional.

DC: That's a good point. That she should have gone the traditional way.

Audience: But it's retrograde. So she wouldn't do it at first.

DC: I don't know if it would have saved her life if she had done something sooner. That's a good point that Saturn is traditional.

Audience: Mars is rising in Capricorn. Sometimes it can be something that is painful, and you will resist but you will gain something from it.

Michael Landon

DC: Yes, for awhile she was improving.

We have been talking about Mars Neptune combinations and I wanted to point out this combination in the 8th house of the chart of Michael Landon. He died of cancer of the pancreas. The eighth house as far as I am concerned can be drastic issues and the potential for a crisis if you have an emphasis there. Now, here's a health crisis. And there's that Mars Neptune again but also Pluto opposite the Ascendant with Michael Landon which can be a difficult transformation in terms of health.

Audience: Does Libra rule the pancreas?

DC: No, Libra rules the kidneys and Virgo rules the function of the pancreas. The pancreas produces hormones to regulate glucose production in the body. Earlier I said I believed Mercury was involved with hormones and Mercury rules Virgo. And if you look at the signs in relation to anatomy, with Aries being the head, Taurus the throat, etc. then Virgo falls where the pancreas is located between the stomach and the spine. I always like to mention that I have not been to medical school. I can't explain a lot of processes in the body. I've learned about the body in terms of medical astrology. I tried to study an anatomy book. If you really want to be a good medical astrologer, you would need to go to med school.

PREDICTIONS

Now, we'll look at transits and some examples. Needless to say, the rules work. The station of a planet on a point in your chart is more difficult that if the planet is moving quickly. So we're talking now about severity and duration of disease. Stations. Eclipses. Transits to the ruler of your chart. These can all affect your health. Looking first at the natal chart, the significators of diseases work. There are astrological significators of diseases, and if you see that you're prone to a disorder and these significators are set off predictive-wise, that's when something can occur.

In terms of predictions you can even work with progressed stationary planets to see if there is an influence in your chart. You can look at your progressed Moon to see your energy levels. You can see if the progressed Moon is hitting anything in your progressed chart or natal chart. Obviously, if your progressed Moon is trining your natal Sun you should be feeling pretty good. If the progressed Moon is squaring your natal Sun, you could be feeling a little down or have less vitality. If your progressed Moon is conjuncting or squaring Saturn, you could be having a problem with teeth or bones; anything like that. Health issues depend on the nature of the planet. So you can look at your progressions.

In terms of transits, the slower the motion the more prolonged the effect of the transiting planet. That's pretty obvious. I would only look at the transiting Sun for a couple of issues. When it's opposite itself it seems to be a low point in the year. Some astrologers say that the month before your solar return can be a low point. I do recall having a very bad day at the dentist, without noticing the transit beforehand, when the transiting Sun was conjunct my natal Saturn – a one-day transit. So when you're planning things, you can look at your Sun for one day – to have a better doctor's appointment, for example.

Mercury is tension or worry, nervous system problems or respiratory system problems. So you could have Mercury hitting your Saturn and maybe for a few days you don't feel very well such as getting an attack of bronchitis or a sore throat. It shouldn't be anything really long lasting from the inner planets. Mercury transit to Saturn is not going to have the severity as Saturn transit is to Mercury, for example. So obviously keep things in perspective. When Venus is transiting you might have a relapse of a condition. I still don't think Venus transits are that difficult except we might eat too much and get indigestion. Also a lack of tone or a need for exercise.

You need to be aware of Mars, especially transiting to the Ascendant. See where it is transiting in your chart. You can have an accident; you are more accident-prone with Mars aspecting your Ascendant or your Sun or even Mars to Mars. It stirs things up. Tension. Stress. Carelessness. Tripping on something in your own home or falling. These are all Mars transits.

Jupiter is associated with excess and congestion. Weight gain. If you have a lot of difficult aspects in your chart by transit and Jupiter is also involved, it's possible it could make a situation worse. I have seen it help in most cases. My best example is a friend who got cancer and the day she started chemotherapy and radiation, Jupiter went over her Ascendant. And then the day she finished the therapy, Jupiter went into her second house. I just thought that was fascinating. And she's fine. It was 15 years ago that she had stomach cancer. So that was a really helpful case of Jupiter. At other times Jupiter may not be so helpful. It could expand a difficult situation.

Saturn teaches us lessons. If you've been ignoring your physical body and you get a difficult Saturn transit, and again I should probably use the words to the personal points – the Sun, Moon, Ascendant, and MC, you could get a lesson in terms of health. Something that's going to restrict you, something chronic, something hardening, a disability, depletion, deposits in the body, cramps or chills. All of these are Saturnine. I believe if you have an arthritic problem, it will start acting up under a Saturn transit. The same with problems with the bones or joints. Avoid getting a chill during a difficult Saturn transit.

Uranus is related to the nervous system. Both Mercury and Uranus are associated with the nervous system. Uranus is more difficult. It's a spasm, a seizure, a heart attack. Usually it's Sun, Mars and Uranus in aspect for a heart attack.

Audience: I have seen so many times with Uranus with the Moon in some aspect to be stomach problems.

DC: You've seen it with Uranus. I've seen it with Mars also – stomach problems. You could get a really nervous disorder with Uranus. Mars Moon can be an indication of ulcers if it shows up in a natal chart, but it can also be digestive problems in general. Uranus, like Mars, could be accidents.

Neptune – a greater tendency to disease and infection. Misdiagnosis. Diseases difficult to diagnose, not recognizing that you even have a problem, deep-seated problems, drug or alcohol related problems, etc.

Pluto – transformation of health patterns and diet. Surgery, hidden transformations in the body that suddenly emerge, reproductive problems, endocrine gland problems, hereditary problems, an abortion, an abnormal growth. These are all related to Pluto. A benign growth would be Venus; a malignant growth would be Plutonian.

Audience: Hysterectomy?

DC: A hysterectomy – Moon Mars or Moon Uranus seems to show up for that. An affliction to the Moon usually.

PREDICTIONS IN ACTION

Audience: Do you generally use transiting midpoints?

DC: I've used the transiting midpoint ephemeris, and occasionally I look at transiting midpoints but not in every case. Most astrological programs can generate transiting midpoints. To a certain extent we didn't need any more information on some charts, as it is very obvious that something is going on. In cases such as Jackie Kennedy Onassis, knowing specific dates, the transiting midpoints can give more information. The announcement that she had Non-Hodgkin's lymphoma was in January 1994. That month Saturn/Pluto by transit = MC by sesquiquadrate. Even more difficult was she had been getting Saturn transit opposite natal Neptune that can be a serious health concern.

Robert Urich was diagnosed in 1996 with cancer. We did his midpoints earlier. And he had Saturn transit square Uranus, Saturn transit square Mars, and I thought this was an interesting one – the progressed Neptune squaring the progressed Midheaven and the progressed Midheaven squaring natal Neptune – all in the same year.

Audience: Can you repeat that again?

DC: He had progressed Neptune square progressed Midheaven on October 7, 1996. And during the same month progressed Midheaven was squaring natal Neptune. He had the progressed Midheaven in Cancer. He had a Mars trine Neptune progression to progression. Now for awhile he was recovering. And he also had Jupiter on the day of surgery applying to his Vertex. So I thought he had a pretty good chance to overcome the illness. The day of his operation the Moon was applying to Jupiter. He was operated on Nov. 14, 1996. When you look at his chart you see some helpful influences, and it doesn't hurt to have Jupiter coming to the Vertex. Because this was after his surgery and this is how astrology is supposed to help us by seeing what is coming up. Robert Urich did recover for a time. (See Chapter Ten, "Tools in Medical Astrology" for more information on the use of eclipses in prediction using the charts of Robert Urich and Carl Sagan.)

Audience: You were talking about the Mars/Neptune midpoint. Can it be anywhere in the chart or does it matter?

DC: For planets angular houses are stronger. Midpoints are not usually read alone so the house position shouldn't matter. What matters is if Mars/Neptune equals a personal point. Or you can take the organ ruled by the sign at the Mars/Neptune midpoint as a weak or toxic point in the body. In Jackie Kennedy Onassis's chart we saw Neptune and Mars both elevated and even though they weren't conjunct, they still stood out. This combination can also describe notoriety. I also have her other midpoints, but the difficult midpoints in her chart could also describe her involvement in the Kennedy assassination. That was a pretty dreadful thing. She could have been shot also. So you don't know that it's going to manifest as health, and she had some difficult midpoints. I would say a square of Mars to Neptune is a difficult combination.

I wasn't planning on going through all the aspects as there's too many, but I would like to add to what I said about Mars and Saturn because of the Mars/Saturn midpoint and the nature of Mars and Saturn. I mentioned looking to see which one is stronger in your chart because you can experience inflammation if Mars is stronger as far as the kinds of diseases you get, and you can have stiffness if Saturn is stronger. Saturn is associated with rheumatic problems and Mars with blood ailments. Mars Neptune aspects can be difficult, but so can a Mars Saturn aspect. I would build up minerals in the body if you have a difficult Mars Saturn aspect. You may be anemic. You may have an iron deficiency; that sort of thing. I would build up the adrenals if you've got a problem with Mars Neptune or Mars Saturn because these aspects can lead to adrenal insufficiency. Needless to say you need to see a nutritionist or a medical doctor for proper treatment.

Years ago I heard that anyone who has a really serious disease had a less serious disease earlier in the life. It is sort of a warning. So I would heed that part of the body that is weak and know that it could get worse later in life. Most problems get worse the older you get. Problems such as broken bones are Mars Saturn. Blocked energy also.

Mars Uranus combinations can indicate surgery, but it's also nervous stress. With a Mars Uranus aspect there's the potential for stomach disorders; you may not be able to tolerate highly spiced food. The same thing if you have a Moon Uranus or a Moon Mars hard aspect. There are foods you can eat or should not eat if you know your aspects. There are vitamins and minerals you can take. I also use homeopathic remedies. I don't think homeopathic remedies can cure cancer, but I think they can nip certain illnesses in the bud. I think they are helpful and deserve further study. And there are also herbs. I mentioned earlier that I went from six colds a year to none in ten years just by changing my diet and taking vitamins. And I didn't take a lot of vitamins, and I didn't do anything radical. It wasn't as if I never ate another French fry or a potato chip. I just believe that if 80% of what you put into you body is good for you, then you can have 20% junk food. That's my motto for myself anyway. And it works for me. But don't have 80% junk food and a carrot once a week and wonder why your body is falling apart.

Basically, you put the planets together to see if they are going to help you or hurt you. Usually a Sun Jupiter combination is going to help you, but at its worst you are going to overeat and become obese or get gout – that sort of thing or become highly toxic. So you look to your aspects to see how well they mesh. Sun Saturn – dental problems – usually it's a square or a hard aspect. Sun Saturn shows up with people who have bulimia or anorexia. Saturn in the fourth house seems to show up in eating disorders also. You can also look at the planets in the houses for more information – for example, Mars or Pluto rising. Overdoing it. The body breaks down because it can't handle any more stress. Being a workaholic. Never taking a break. The man who had Lou Gehrig's disease who had Mars rising told me he never stopped for a second. And now he's in a wheelchair. The chart has warnings and you should heed them. Your body can just take so much or it will break down. Sun Uranus – spasm conditions, cold sweats. I think Sun Uranus has to do with being affected by weather changes; the changes in the barometer can affect your moods or even vitality. Sun Neptune can also be vitality problems as well as allergies, fluid imbalance, eye problems and sometimes a weak heart. Sun Pluto – pushing yourself to the limit. Similar to Pluto rising.

Audience: Do you use the inconjunct?

DC: I use the inconjunct as a difficult aspect between planets. So, yes, I do use it. I just take a sheet of paper and I start listing significators. Let's say I'm looking for a particular problem in the chart. I make a list of the significators in the chart and if the list has lots of significators for a particular problem, then I decide that the person has a weakness in that area of the body or a proneness to a specific disease. If I only see a couple of things I consider it borderline, and I say it's a part of the body that could be problematic if you neglect it. You evaluate your list of significators such as for respiratory or blood sugar problems to see where there is weakness in the body.

Audience: If you see problems in the body, do you time them by solar arc or transit?

DC: Yes and no. Again, you have to be careful. You can't always be sure how the predictions will manifest. I think you can look and say that I'd better get more rest. I'm getting a Saturn transit. I'd better take more minerals. I think you can do it that way. Why would you want to know? Oh, next year I'm going to get sick. I don't use it like that. I think you can use the information to take the right vitamins and herbs or prepare yourself for periods of stress.

1   This book is available and has recently been reprinted.

2   Davidson, William: *Davidson's Medical Astrology,* Astrological Bureau, Monroe, New York, 1979.

3   Starck, Marcia, *Astrology Key to Holistic Health,* Seek-It Publications, Birmingham, MI 1982.

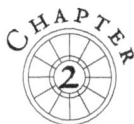

PRACTICAL APPROACHES
TO MEDICAL ASTROLOGY

In Chapter Two you will learn more about the planets in medical astrology in terms of meanings and in combination and how to spot potential health problems. There are more chart examples utilizing the planets and the signs as well as predictive techniques.

There are ways to quickly hone in on potential health problems in the natal chart. Obviously, you're not going to get all the answers without some searching, but some problems are very obvious and some techniques are simple to use such as the elements, which are discussed in Chapter Six: "Rebalancing with the Elements and Modes." Some techniques are not so easy to use, and that's when you have to sit down and do a lot of research. The purpose of this chapter is to show what can be seen quickly in a chart to point out a potential health problem.

Noel Tyl has written a medical astrology book[1] describing how you can look ahead and use predictions as you say to yourself, "Maybe I should get a checkup; I've got some difficult transits coming." Why wait until you've got difficult transits or directions when you can start looking at your chart at as young an age as you want to evaluate your strengths and weaknesses. You can do this with medical astrology. Once you discover a weakness, you can see what measures you can take to strengthen that part of the body. If you don't have enough fire, for example, then incorporate techniques that increase fire. (See Chapter Six for a discussion of the elements.)

I always like to give some disclaimers when I am talking about medical astrology. Number 1. I am not a physician, and I get very confused myself on anatomy and physiology even though I've tried to read books on these subjects. I've never claimed to any client that I have the knowledge of a medical doctor because I don't, and neither should you unless you've been to med school. Number 2. You have to be very careful of what you tell people. You can see the most difficult planetary configurations in a chart, but you don't know for sure how they will manifest. It may not be health related. It could be something with real estate, a job, a marriage. I have to say that when the Ascendant is involved it has a lot to do with health. The more I look at health, the more I find the Ascendant is involved – the 1 – 7 axis. However, in general, use medical astrology more to see what kind of strengths and weaknesses show up in the chart as well as potential treatment options and periods of stress.

As mentioned briefly in Chapter One, when you are looking at a chart the weakest point is considered the sign anatomically related to the sign Saturn occupies. Where there is a rich blood supply you are nourished in that part of the body. Where there is a lesser blood supply, that is where you are weakened and that is where Saturn falls in your chart. So that's one of the first things you should be thinking of when you look at your chart and you ask yourself what part of my body could be weak? Where is Saturn in my chart by sign? And because the crosses work in medical astrology, if you have Saturn in a fixed sign, you can have a weakness in the whole fixed cross. I find it's usually the sign that Saturn is in or the sign opposite that is the weakest. So if you have Saturn in Taurus, you can find that your weakness is either in Taurus or Scorpio. It could also be a weakness in one of the other fixed signs – Leo or Aquarius.

The planets were discussed in Chapter One. To reiterate it is the planets in combination with each other that define the problems. The planets in combination with each other along with the signs and houses are the disease indicators in the chart. The Sun rules vitality, but if the Sun is receiving a hard aspect from, for example, Saturn or Neptune, then the action of the Sun is compromised. So you know right away, you could have a vitality problem or you also could be more prone to infection. Because an afflicted Sun generally shows up as energy problems or a fever or inflammation.

Audience: What if you have a hard aspect with Neptune but a good aspect with Mars?

DC: If the Mars is well aspected, it will help a lot. You probably could still get infections, but they won't be as serious or as long lasting since you have the help from Mars. If something in your chart compensates for a difficult aspect, it doesn't mean you won't ever get ill because everybody gets sick at some point in their life. The duration and the severity of the illness will be modified by the planets that counteract the difficult aspects. And then you can sit down and see what is coming up over the course of time and see if you have some difficult transits or directions.

Lunar problems have to do with fluids in the body, discharges. It's the female cycle. It has to do with mucous formation, water retention. Mercury seems to definitely show up with respiratory or nervous system disorders. And Mercury is involved with the hormones. As mentioned, Pluto is the whole endocrine system in the body, but the messages or the hormones have to do with Mercury. Mercury is also mental disorders, nervous disorders –that sort of thing. Venus has to do with a lack of tone in your body. Neptune has to do with a lack of tone also. Earlier I said that where Saturn falls in your chart is the weakest point in your body. Well, where Neptune falls there can be a weakness too. It's another part of the body you need to build up. Venus shows up with blood sugar problems. Venus rules sugar; Jupiter rules fat. You can think of it that way. Venus rules the veins. Jupiter rules the arteries. That is why Jupiter Saturn combinations show up as arteriosclerosis. And Venus Saturn problems show up as phlebitis. This is the difference. This is where you can start to see how the aspects combine. Jupiter Saturn problems also can be liver or gallbladder disorders but basically can be arteriosclerosis since Jupiter rules the arteries. But phlebitis, because Venus rules the veins, is a Venus Saturn problem because Saturn is keeping the Venus from doing its job. By the way, lately I have been using the 22½ degree aspect and finding amazing things with it. You know that's half of the 45-degree aspect. I didn't use it for years but now thanks to computer programs you can set your computer to list it. A friend of mine who had a liver transplant had an exact 22½ degree aspect between Jupiter and Saturn. Saturn restricts the function of the liver – Jupiter. Use it only if it's almost exact – like up to a 30" orb.

Audience: What about the midpoint?

DC: Well, the midpoint is something else. Possibly if the Sun = Jupiter/Saturn it would have a similar meaning. Now the aspect was Jupiter 22½ degrees to Saturn. The symbol looks like the semi-square with a line drawn through it.

Audience: Do you find it works in transits?

DC: I have looked at the 22½ degree aspect briefly in transits, and it does work but you can get overwhelmed with too much information. We are already printing out reams of paper with all the techniques we can do with computers.

Venus is benign growths. Saturn is not so benign. Your skin cancer is going to be shown by Saturn which rules the skin, but skin problems that don't lead to serious disease are ruled by Venus. I always like to show a contrast between planets. Mars is infection, but Pluto is massive infection. Venus rules the skin, but it is more cosmetic problems. Saturn is much more difficult in relation to the skin.

Audience: Can Saturn have to do with tumors?

DC: Saturn can be tumors but so can Neptune and Pluto. Unfortunately, I have a lot of cancer cases, and there is no way to totally describe all the significators for cancer. Saturn is hardening, but so are fixed signs. So it's not that simple.

So the venous circulation of the body is ruled by Venus and also the idea of balance in the body. For example, if you have an afflicted Venus you could be the type who always bumps into things. Mars is infection and inflammation. It's on a higher level than the Sun where Pluto is the highest of them all in terms of infection. Mars is bruises; it's surgery; it's wounds; it's burns; it's blood.

Audience: Would you say Mars is accidents?

DC: Yes, it also rules accidents. That's Mars for sure. Also Uranus. Sexual dysfunction can show up with Mars also.

Jupiter, again, diseases caused by excess, fatty degeneration. If you have a problem with fat assimilation, and that could be shown by Saturn in Sagittarius or any Jupiter Saturn in hard aspect that's something else you should be aware of – how you assimilate fats. Because if we are what we eat, not 100%, but food is the fuel that keeps us going, and you lack fire so you're not digesting your food properly or you have a Jupiter Saturn issue and you're not digesting fats properly – these can all lead to health problems. Or you have a Venus problem and the sugar metabolism isn't right. You can see simplistic things in a chart and then you can take it a step further to see a doctor, nutritionist or another heath professional. This kind of information gets you started. I have seen Jupiter save people's lives and I have seen Jupiter end people's lives. I still think it's a beneficial planet. I hear astrologers say it does all these awful things but I don't agree. I think most of the time it's going to save you.

Saturn, as we said, is crystallization, hardening, chronic disease, also deafness. It's alkaline where Mars is acidic. It's chronic weakness, it's the skeleton in our body, our teeth. It denotes stoppage. With Saturn there can be under activity, blockages. And it's also involved with dental problems and malnutrition. Again, it's Saturn in combination. Saturn in Cancer or Saturn in the fourth house can indicate anorexia, problems with the stomach or food assimilation. So you have to take these keywords a step further.

Uranus is spasms, seizure, shock, cramps, anything unusual or twisted in the body, also sudden illness.

As discussed in Chapter One, Neptune is the most difficult of all the planets as far as medical astrology is concerned. A disease just creeps up on you. It's considered the most difficult and insidious of all the planets. It can be poisoning, hidden illness, misdiagnosis, problems with the immune system – especially a Mars Neptune combination for lowered immune function. Also Neptune for drug addiction, lack of tone. It deceives you, it hides, it disguises.

Pluto can describe genetic problems, abnormal growths. Procedures like amputations are Plutonian. Malformation, birth defects, anything drastic is Pluto.

Audience: In order for it to happen, you have to have it in your natal chart?

DC: Right. What I've done just now is given you keywords for the planets, how they work in medical astrology. You have to use the planets in combination and learn the significators of various diseases and then see if you have these significators in your own natal chart.

For example, when the Sun is in hard aspect with the Moon you may have eye problems or vitality problems. Unless there's something really malefic in your chart, you're not going to be blind from this combination. You just may need glasses. You have to be aware – what does this planet rule? The Sun rules Leo which is associated with the heart and the back. If Saturn or Neptune, for example, squares your Sun, you may have heart problems or back problems. You have to combine all the aspects in the chart; you don't always know how they will manifest. Don't diagnose with medical astrology. Even Reinhold Ebertin, who was a cosmobiologist and a prolific writer on medical astrology advises not to diagnose with medical astrology at the beginning of his book, *Astrological Healing The History And Practice Of Astromedicine*[3]. Medical astrology is to help you confirm things or to see what is coming up. You can take the chart apart and you can see your strengths and weaknesses, but somebody cannot call you on the phone and ask if you can tell them what's wrong with them. And if you try to diagnose and you're not a doctor, you're breaking the law.

Now, I want to give some chart examples. In Chapter One the chart of a woman diagnosed with breast cancer was discussed in reference to the planets Mars and Neptune. Another Mars Neptune example is the chart labeled ALS which is Lou Gehrig's disease. This is another example of angular planets. The angles are where the potency is and where you can immediately spot potential problems. And the Ascendant can represent the physical body. The Sun I believe is more your vitality and how you ward off disease although it does have to do with health. There's something about the Ascendant when if it's affected, for example, by an eclipse or an outer planet transit that you had better pay attention to your body. I also think the Ascendant is your immediate environment too where things can change. It's definitely associated with health.

Both the breast cancer chart and ALS chart have Mars rising. The ALS chart has a mundane square. (Larousse[4] defines it as an aspect measured along the celestial equator, in Right Ascension, as distinguished from a zodiacal aspect, which is measured along the ecliptic, in Celestial

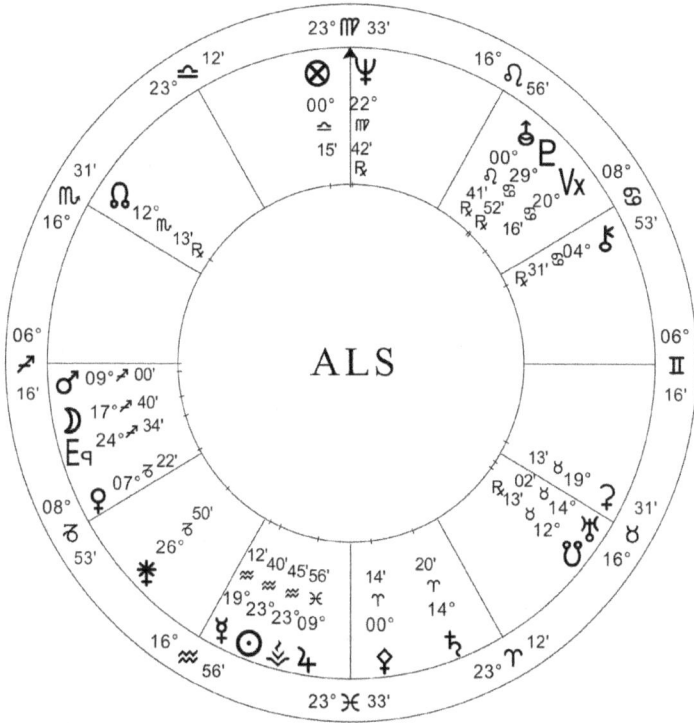

Longitude.) Mars conjunct the Ascendant and Neptune conjunct the MC are in mundane square to each other. It is also called in mundo. If you have planets that are conjunct angles but are not necessarily in aspect to each other in longitude, they can act like a square. This ALS chart has Mars rising. He did tell me he burned himself out. People who have Mars rising don't know how to stop. You'd better take a break or slow down because maybe mentally you don't notice it, but your body does, and you really can become debilitated over the course of time.

The ALS chart is a case of Neptune afflicting Mars by mundane square as I wanted you to be aware of that type of aspect. The breast cancer chart was an example of a square of Mars to Neptune. Both charts have an elevated Neptune. I wanted to throw in the signs to see if we can see a difference in diseases. Why did one person get Lou Gehrig's disease and another get breast cancer? I don't think you can really answer it except to say that Sagittarius is a sign of locomotion and you lose your ability to get around when you get Lou Gehrig's disease as it just gets worse and worse. (I also have this case discussed in more detail in my book *How To Give An Astrological Health Reading*[5].) Here's a case (ALS) where a sign of locomotion shows up. Now the breast cancer chart with Capricorn rising is opposite Cancer in the zodiac which is the cardinal sign which rules the breasts. So in a way the charts did point out why one got Lou Gehrig's disease and the other got breast cancer. It's never that simple, and it's easier in retrospect.

I wanted to give an example on how the signs sometimes point out the specifics of a disease with the planets being the major game players.

Audience: If you are looking at a child's chart and you see these types of difficulties and you say to the parents, I see blah, blah, blah, how much can you mitigate that Mars Neptune by cleansing certain things in the body and using herbs or supplements?

DC: Unfortunately, that's a question that no one can really answer. There's nothing like starting young, working on your body and taking care of your body especially knowing there can be a weakness in the immune system. You could utilize the sign of your Mars/Neptune midpoint also as a weak point in the body and build it up. Also Mars Neptune combinations can be artistic or musical so you want to allow for creative growth.

Audience: How do you deal with conjunctions to personal planets?

DC: I'm going to show you three charts with Jupiter Saturn conjunctions and describe what happened to each individual. The conjunctions are difficult if it's an outer planet to an inner planet. Though I think squares are more difficult than conjunctions, an outer planet conjunction to a personal point can be stressful.

Audience: In response to what you said, I had a child who had five outer planets retrograde diagnosed with cerebral palsy and using certain health regimes has improved each and every year and is doing phenomenally well today.

DC: So you can do things to improve a difficult chart.

Audience: I'd like to address the question about improving the immune system. There are certain things you can do. There are combinations of herbs that can help. Astragalus can help. There are some mushrooms that can help. You can use Neptune in a positive way. The other thing is about the sensitivity. Somebody could be a great musician. I really think it's comes down to that sensitivity and how it is used or misused. Because it's that sensitivity that is able to translate their experience and make it something that everybody can empathize with. But it's also when that sensitivity, when it's hypersensitive and they can't deal with their pain; they run away from it. They look for an escape.

DC: Right, possibly by using drugs. I remember that Ingrid Naiman mentioned lotus root for the adrenals.

Audience: I have to ask since you mentioned music, but there are some people who are sensitive to sound where music can automatically unblock them.

DC: Yes, that's one cure.

Let's look at the three examples of a Jupiter Saturn conjunction. Look at the chart labeled Throat Disorder – Jupiter Saturn conjunction in Taurus on the Ascendant. The Ascendant is the body and of course it's a personal point. Taurus is the throat. It's a case of throat cancer. He's fine but he did have throat cancer. The next chart – Bi-polar Disorder- has a Jupiter Saturn conjunction in Libra on the Midheaven – another personal point. This person was diagnosed with a bi-polar mental disease. Isn't it interesting that this conjunction is in Libra (kidneys) that are involved in excreting wastes from the body and the homeostasis balance in the body? Maybe this individual has a chemical imbalance that can be helped by medicine or diet. I thought it was interesting how the Jupiter Saturn showed up in that chart.

Audience: Libra is opposite Aries that has to do with the brain.

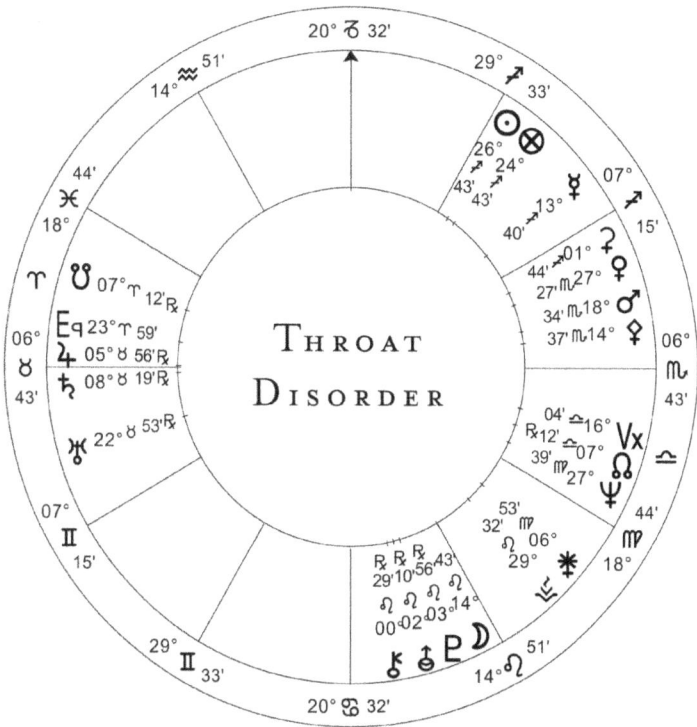

THROAT DISORDER

DC: Good point.

The third Jupiter Saturn example I wanted you to see is labeled Quadruple Bypass. Notice this chart has a Mars Neptune conjunction and a Jupiter Saturn conjunction that is connected to the Mars Neptune conjunction by sesquiquadrate. Jupiter rules the Ascendant. Now what house is the Jupiter Saturn conjunction in?

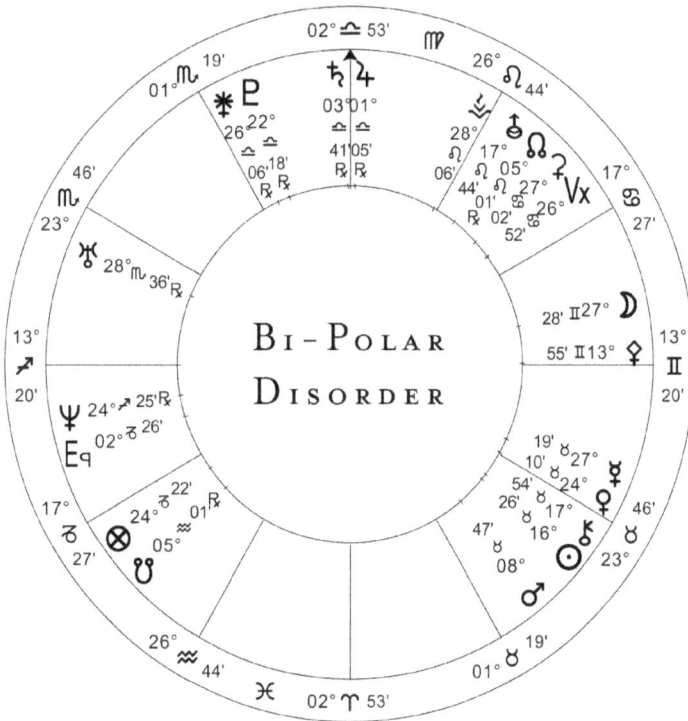

B I - P O L A R
D I S O R D E R

Audience: The fifth house.

DC: And does the fifth house tell you anything?

Audience: The heart.

DC: Right. He had quadruple bypass surgery. Now here's a case of the fixed cross with both Jupiter and Saturn in Taurus. With Jupiter Saturn combinations, which I've said earlier, Saturn restricts Jupiter which rules fats and fat assimilation and the arteries. And then it's connected to the fifth house. Malefics in the fifth house are a signature of heart disease and it's the fixed cross. This is the Taurus, Scorpio, Leo, Aquarius, heart and circulation cross of the body, and in this case shows that it could be something that affects the heart.

Audience: It's a Libra Sun sign and Venus is in Leo in mutual reception to the Sun and square the Jupiter Saturn. The Leo being the heart.

DC: Right. But it's a very wide square. I'm not going into deep interpretation on these charts. I'm using them more to point things out.

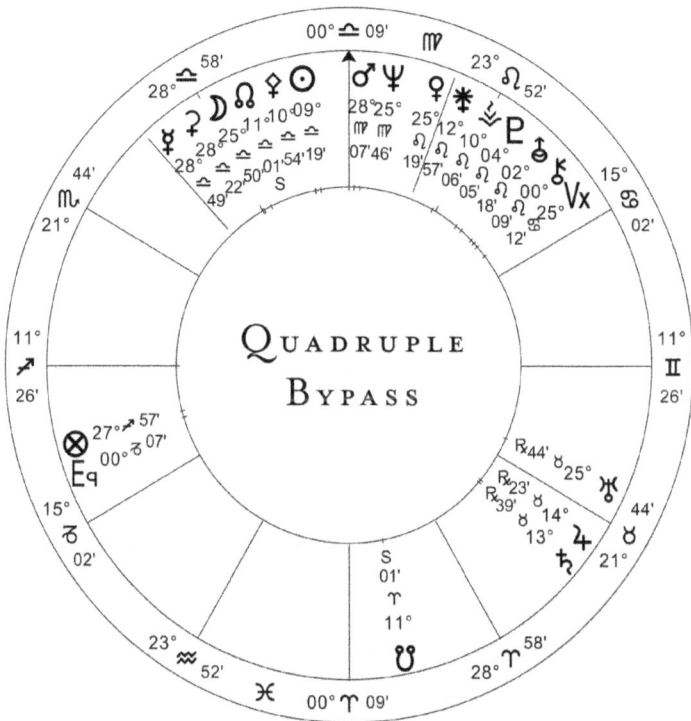

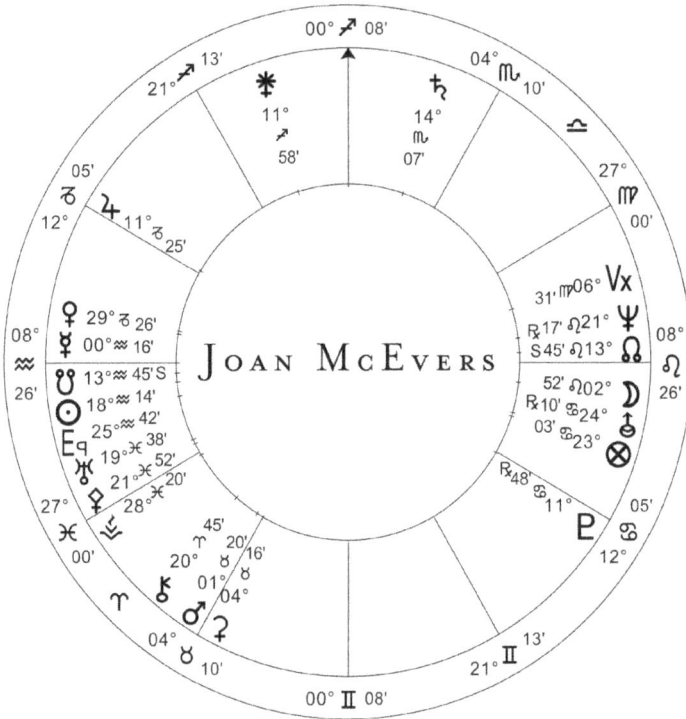

Audience: The Jupiter Saturn is retrograde. Does that make a difference?

DC: Supposedly, retrogrades are more difficult in medical astrology. So, it could be more difficult, but so many people are born with this aspect that it's not that simple. I know this person and he never took that great care of himself. He was overweight, etc. and had lots of health problems that could be the Mars Neptune conjunction. I just thought that here were charts where the signs pointed out what happened which was interesting, because I always found

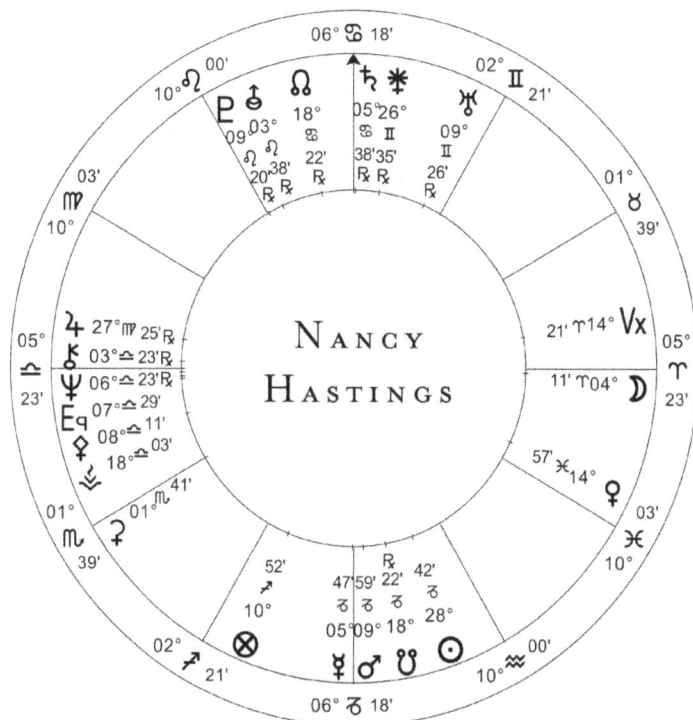

06° ♋ 18'

00'
10° ♌
02° Ⅱ 21'

♇ 09°03° ↑ ♋ 18° ♌ 22' 20°38' ℞ ♌ ℞ ☌ 05°26' ♋ Ⅱ 38'35' ℞ ℞ ♄ ✳ ♅ 09° Ⅱ 26° ℞

03' ♍ 10°

01° ♉ 39'

05° ♎ 23' ♃ 27°♍25'℞ ⚷ 03°♎23'℞ ♆ 06°♎23'℞ ☄ 07°♎29' ♀ 08°♎11' 18°♎03'

NANCY
HASTINGS

21' ♈14° Vx
11' ♈04° ☽

05° ♈ 23'

01° ♏ 39' ☌ 01°♏41' ⚹ 57' ♓14°

03' ♓ 10°

02° ♐ 21' ⊗ 52' 10° ♐ 47'59' ℞ ☿ ♂ ☊ ☉ 22' 42' ♑ ♑ ♑ ♑ 05°09° 18° 28° 10° ♒ 00'

06° ♑ 18'

the hardest part of medical astrology is to fit the signs in with everything else. These were good examples, but again it's easier in retrospect.

We will look at Nancy Hastings' chart (also referred to in "Rebalancing with the Elements and the Modes") and Joan McEvers' chart. McEvers had a stroke. What I thought was fascinating was what happened with Joan McEvers' progressed planets. Now the first thing that you can see when you look at Joan McEvers chart is a first house Sun. We have the first house that is the physical body and added to that the Sun. And I have a few charts of people with first house Sun's who had brain tumors. And they didn't have any planets in Aries. There's something about the first house being the natural house of Aries that is associated with the brain. When you look at a chart, the houses can show an emphasis and in this case the first house being the natural house of Aries is associated with strokes. Her Mars is in Taurus. So what does that tell you about the capabilities of her Mars? Mars is the old ruler of Scorpio. Don't forget the old rulers. Mars therefore is in detriment in Taurus. Jupiter used to rule Pisces. Saturn ruled Aquarius. They all count in medical astrology. So Mars is in detriment. It's not working up to its full potential as far as being able to fight. Remember Mars is your fight in your chart.

Audience: Mohammed Ali has Mars in Taurus.

DC: Well, he used it as a fighter but look at how ill he is today.

The Sun in the first house is afflicted. So we know there is a first house problem. And the Sun equals the Saturn/Neptune midpoint and it's an indirect midpoint. What I thought was so interesting when she had her stroke, she had three planets progress into Aries in the 12th house of her progressed chart. The stroke was September 4, 1995, but I felt we should also be looking at the progressed chart. She had Venus, Mercury and the Sun all at the end of Aries when she had her stroke all falling in the 12th house of the progressed chart. So I thought it was very interesting as it was a whole Aries phenomena and a first house problem natally which brings us to one other point.

If you have natal planets in the 11th and 12th houses as in Scot Hamilton's chart (also discussed in "Rebalancing with the Elements and Modes"), by solar arc they are going to hit your Ascendant at some point in your life. I got his chart from Noel Tyl's book *(Astrological Timing of Critical Illness)*. And Noel Tyl goes into a lot more detail on Scott Hamilton's early life and how he was very ill as a child which is why he only grew to be 5'3". So there's a lot more to Scott Hamilton's medical history than we're doing now, but he did get testicular cancer.

In his book Tyl discusses solar arcs and also the occurrence of Sun Pluto aspects. I have found they can be in longitude or in declination. When I started looking at these charts I did see Sun Pluto combinations in some of them. And they all had difficult health problems. So

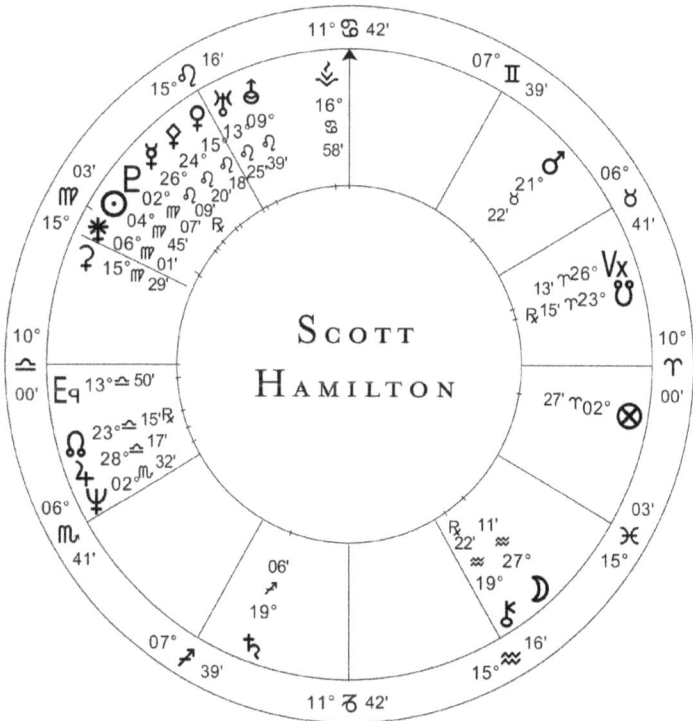

SCOTT HAMILTON

that's another aspect to be aware of for health problems. In Scott Hamilton's chart, Pluto came to his Ascendant by solar arc at the time when he got ill. And he has Sun conjunct Pluto. So be aware of your planets moving by solar arc toward your Ascendant if you have difficult planets coming out of your 11th or 12th houses. That's something else that's easy to spot.

Audience: Do you look at the 6th house?

DC: I would look at the sixth house if the Sun were there.

Audience: What if Neptune were there?

DC: If Neptune were there, I might think you had allergies.

Audience: Misdiagnosis?

DC: Yes, and misdiagnosis. In terms of medical astrology the sixth house and the 12th house show up in illness but an emphasized sixth or 12th house shows up in the charts of health care workers also. I know many people who work in hospitals have planets in the 12th house.

Look at Nancy Hastings' chart. She wrote two astrology books on progressions and died in 1991. She was quite a well-known and renown astrologer and her books are excellent. This is an example of all the angles being afflicted and a person with severe health problems. The strongest and the most difficult problems can be a result of malefics on the angles. So this is an example of the planets in action in a negative way because you can see that grand cross on the angles in cardinal signs and she died from cancer. Mars is opposite Saturn and square Neptune with the involvement of the Moon. Here is where the Mars does not get to work at its best.

If you see this in your chart, or Mars in Pisces, you've got to do something to build up your immune system. You should find any information you can on building up the adrenals and the immune system to fight off disease. For good vitality you need a strong Sun and a strong Mars and probably a strong Jupiter and a decent amount of fire in your chart for fight. Because what is fight but your body burning off toxins or resisting disease. And what is the burning – it's the fevers you get. The fevers that you get are shown by the fire in a chart or aspects involving the Sun or Mars. Fevers burn off toxins.

What can you say to someone with a chart like this? She was an astrologer. She knew she had this chart. This chart was in Lee Lehman's Classical Astrology book[6]. I'm sure it made her a hard worker and a good writer as she used the energy that way.

Audience: She had Neptune on the rising square the MC which was her closest aspect which is what made her an astrologer, but with Neptune on the rising you can't see frequently what's in front of you.

DC: Yes, that's a good point. And what if you know all this astrological information? What can you do about it? I think to a certain extent be very rigorous in regards to health if you know you have a difficult chart. Look, I'm going to have to be very disciplined during my life. And sure I'd like to eat all this junk food. But I'd better avoid it. I'm reading the biography of Andy Kaufman written by his best friend. He died of cancer while in his early 30's. Apparently, he was a chocoholic and lived on chocolate. And when he was dying he said something like "the

61

chocolate killed me." So I don't think diet saves you 100% but I certainly think it helps.

Audience: In answer to your question, what can you say to a person, you can say to a person that anyone can overcome their chart. My daughter has all these problems and has Neptune in the 6th and it affected her blood and the iron levels and she was very deficient that way. But through replacement over time she was able to more than overcome her chart.

DC: You have a positive attitude that you can overcome your chart. I know some astrologers who think that everything is fate and that's it. If you see someone and their adrenal system shows up as weak in their chart, you can say that if I were you I would do such and such. Point clients in a helpful direction either to useful books or a health practitioner. Not that's it. There's nothing you can do. I've heard terrible things that astrologers have said to people.

If you have a well-aspected Sun you can overcome a lot. If you have a strong Mars, you can overcome a lot. If not, do what you can to build up the Solar energy and the Martian energy.

Audience: Pluto opposing the Sun. Would that help recuperation?

DC: Pluto opposing the Sun can be difficult. Ingrid Naiman talks about Moon Pluto people harming their adrenals because of all the extra fight. Pluto is sometimes always ready for a fight. And some of these difficult charts as I told you had Sun Pluto aspects. Look at your parallels too when you're checking aspects.

One chart – the breast cancer chart discussed in Chapter One – had the Sun opposite Pluto. Scott Hamilton had the Sun conjunct Pluto. Robert Urich had a Sun Pluto aspect by sesquiquadrate and the throat cancer case had the Sun contra-parallel Pluto. The Bi-Polar example has Sun quincunx Pluto. The Quadruple Bypass case has the Sun sextile Pluto, and he has been able to overcome some rather difficult health problems.

Audience: Pluto doesn't have to manifest that way.

DC: It could be somebody who is a great leader. It can describe a very powerful person.

Audience: When you see these aspects in solar return charts, are you saying this could initiate a health problem?

DC: I recently did a lecture on solar returns and medical astrology, and I was able to see someone who had a hysterectomy that showed up in the solar return. I haven't been using them for health that much, but I think you can see some health problems in solar returns. Since there are so many ways of dong solar returns – some people precess them; some don't. Some do them for the birthplace. Some for the location you are at on your birthday. And some for where they live. I think you're better off sticking with transits, progressions and solar arcs.

You could also use the transiting midpoints and transits to midpoints. You get a lot of answers that way. In my experience the solar return isn't as good for timing as transits, progressions and directions. I use it as an overall outlook for the year.

Audience: ADD?

DC: Oh, attention deficit disorder. That's a Mercury problem.

Audience: Let's say a person has Mercury Neptune conjunct, Mercury Pluto sextile and Mercury Uranus square. Is that a learning disorder?

DC: I've had charts like that with children who had learning disorders. And I noticed there was a retrograde Mercury too with the learning disorders, more than with a direct Mercury.

Audience: Another chart I saw with ADD, this was my ex-husband; he has Mercury Uranus conjunct in Gemini sextile Jupiter in Sagittarius. These charts are also brilliant people.

DC: Everybody learns differently and that's what the chart also shows – how you learn.

1   Tyl, Noel: *Astrological Timing of Critical Illness,* *Llewellyn,* 1998.

2   Starck,Marcia: *Healing with Astrology,* The Crossing Press, 1997.

3   Ebertin, Reinhold: *Astrological Healing The History And Practice Of Astromedicine,* Samuel Weiser, Inc, 1989.

4   Brau, Jean-Louis, Weaver, Helen and Edmands, Allan, *Larousse Encyclopedia of Astrology,* Librairie Larousse, 1977. (pg 193).

5   Cramer, Diane: *How To Give An Astrological Health Reading,* AFA, Tempe, AZ, 1996.

6   Lehman, Ph.D, Dr. J. Lee: *Classical Astrology for Modern Living,* Whitford Press, 1996.

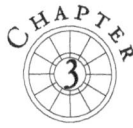

IDENTIFYING HEART DISEASE IN
THE NATAL CHART

This chapter describes in depth the various types of disorders associated with the heart along with the astrological indicators. Chart examples are used to illustrate the astrological significators in action.

This is a complicated subject that takes years to learn, and I doubt many of us are cardiologists. I don't have a total grasp of the subject as I am not a physician, but I do feel I have an understanding of heart disease as seen in a birth chart. So we're going to take a very complex subject and look at it in terms of categories. I'll describe the different types of heart problems and what signifies them astrologically. We will examine the charts of persons with heart disease to illustrate the astrological techniques. This is an important topic since heart disease is considered to be the number one health problem in the United States.

Heart disease can involve other diseases. It can include problems with the kidneys and other organs. So it isn't always the heart causing the primary problem but for our purposes we are just going to talk about the heart.

Congestive heart failure is a term that means that the heart is not pumping enough blood to the body. There are many things that could cause this. For example, it could be the result of a heart attack or problems with the heart valves or due to kidney failure.

There are many types of afflictions that affect the heart such as congenital disease, valve disease, infiltrative disease, tumors, cardiomyopathies (explained below) and coronary artery disease. And then there are non-cardiac functional diseases where the heart action is halted.

THE MEDICAL TERMS

We'll start with heart disease that affects the coronary arteries which is the type you hear the most about. This information is from a CPR manual.

CAD – coronary artery disease – this is your primary cause of heart attacks. It is a blockage of the coronary arteries that supply blood to the heart muscle. The heart muscle is ruled by Leo. I will give you the medical information and then give you the astrological significators. I think you'll have a better comprehension if you understand the medical part. CAD or arteriosclerosis is the gradual build-up of fatty deposits caused mainly by plaque on the artery walls. CAD essentially narrows the artery and decreases or stops blood flow and may be compared to the gradual buildup of lime deposits in a pipe that ultimately plug the pipe completely. Clogged arteries can lead to a heart attack by forming clots. Clots can also travel to the brain and cause a stroke, or if they go to the lungs can cause a pulmonary embolism. Arteriosclerosis can begin developing at an early age.

Now, here's where astrology can help you. If we can figure out if you are prone to heart disease using your chart, and there are ways you can show it, you may discover that you are a person who is prone to hardening of the arteries. The people who appear to be very healthy and end up having a heart attack are the ones who may not have had symptoms of heart disease. They weren't aware of it, and this is what we can show in the chart.

Significant disease may be present in some individuals before age 20. Long before the function of the heart is diminished there may be an asymptomatic period where risk factor modification may halt or even reverse the process of arteriosclerosis.

This is where exercise, right eating and taking care of your body may prevent heart disease from even starting. You don't want to have a heart attack to find out you have a heart problem. This is where medical astrology can help. There are several symptoms of coronary heart disease. The first one is called angina – a pain in the chest that may be relieved by rest and nitroglycerin. This chest pain is caused by a narrowing of the coronary arteries that prevents the delivery of an adequate supply of blood and oxygen to meet the demands of the working heart muscle. Once the demands of the heart muscle are decreased, the pain disappears and a heart attack can be averted.

The next is Ischemia that can lead to a heart attack. It occurs when the demands of the heart muscle for oxygen greatly exceeds the availability. This is usually a result of severe narrowing or complete blockage of a diseased coronary artery and results in infarction which is explained below. The heart itself needs its own supply of blood and oxygen, which is delivered by the coronary arteries, and if an artery becomes ischemic, angina occurs followed by a heart attack.

CONTRIBUTING FACTORS OF A HEART ATTACK

High blood cholesterol

High blood pressure which weakens the vessel walls

Cigarette smoking which reduces cholesterol breakdown and causes constriction of blood vessels

Lack of exercise

Obesity

Acute myocardial infarction means death of a section of the heart muscle due to an inadequate blood supply to that area. This is another term for heart attack. So is coronary and coronary thrombosis, which are also old-fashioned terms for heart attack.

Then there is what's known as "sudden death." "Sudden death" means that a person having a heart attack who goes into cardiac arrest can possibly be saved by getting immediate CPR and getting to a hospital quickly to receive lifesaving "clot busters." These clot busters are only effective for the first few hours of having a heart attack. According to the CPR manual, you have an excellent chance of saving somebody by immediately initiating CPR. This is why they advise people to learn CPR as you have four times the chance of survival. Without CPR clinical death can occur quickly.

Sudden death can occur shortly after the beginning of a heart attack. In this situation the lay public using CPR can be the first link to survival. This is also called the "sudden death syndrome" which many times can be reversed with CPR. Sudden death can be reversible; biological (or clinical death) cannot. Damage from a heart attack treated within an hour or two can be markedly reduced. Obviously, some people will die, but it is possible to save someone's life if they receive immediate help.

ASTROLOGY RULES

Now I'll cover the astrology with what I just gave you medically. I've read and studied almost all the available literature on medical astrology and have used what I have learned to settle on the various significators of diseases. Very few astrologers agree on rulerships for disease and parts of the body. What it comes down to is the anatomy of the body relates to the signs of the zodiac. Leo rules the heart muscle. Physiology is described by the planets – how the muscle works. Therefore, if there are afflictions involving the sign Leo, you may be prone to heart disease. If the Sun is afflicted you may or you may not be depending on how many significators you have for heart disease. The Sun rules Leo.

One rule of medical astrology states if the ruler of a sign is afflicted, there can be a health problem in the location of the sign. Medically speaking, you have to look at the crosses – the cardinal cross, the fixed cross and the mutable cross. And when it comes to heart disease, the fixed cross is emphasized the most often but not always. That's Taurus, Scorpio, Leo and Aquarius.

In medical astrology the polarities work. You can have an emphasis in the sign of Taurus but have a Scorpio problem in your body. You can have an emphasis in Aquarius and it seems like a Leo problem or even a Taurus problem. Medically, you have to forget your traditional astrology rules because in medical astrology the whole cross comes into play. You can't always be sure which sign in the cross will experience a problem, but most of the time when, for example, you see a circulatory problem you will see a difficulty related to the sign Aquarius. Sometimes it is not that simple.

You will find a list of books at the end of this chapter that includes medical astrology and heart disease. There's a chapter on cardiovascular disorders in the Marcia Starck books. She mentions studies describing type A personalities in relation to heart disease who tend to suffer more from high blood pressure. This type can also be very stubborn and hold back their feelings and are very set in their ways. This could cause congestive circulation.

I think that if you see these symptoms in charts – stubbornness, rigidity – they may develop heart disease. They could also develop arthritis. Everything isn't always that simple. The planets can describe certain personality traits also. Fixed disorders have a lot to do with heart disease. Taurus and Scorpio are associated with cleansing and elimination. When the body is congested circulation becomes difficult. And thus the Taurus Scorpio axis is involved as well as the Leo Aquarius axis. If you have a clogged colon (Scorpio), such as Saturn in Scorpio, you may find that toxins get back into the bloodstream and they circulate and it causes the heart to work harder. Whenever you put too much strain on the heart, you are prone to heart disease.

When you read the Davidson book, which are a series of lectures given in the late 1950's, there's a whole discussion about coronary thrombosis being a colon condition. He talks about Uranus in Scorpio which he says causes antipathy, a circulation of toxins into the body and the symptoms would be dizziness and a pain in the back of your neck. He states that Uranus in Scorpio in bad aspect to the Sun or the Moon has to do with coronary heart disease.

The Doris Chase Doane book is full of studies of different diseases. She gave a preliminary study of coronary thrombosis. And she said that heavy afflictions to a planet in Leo or to the Sun, Venus or Jupiter afflicted and Pluto or Neptune prominent and afflicted indicate heart disease.

Uranus rules the electrical system of the heart. Aquarius rules the oxygen circulation of the body. Venus rules the venous circulation – the veins. Jupiter rules arterial circulation – the arteries. Clogging of the arteries can be seen with a Jupiter Saturn affliction or Jupiter in Capricorn or possibly Saturn in Sagittarius. When you have problems involving the veins it will be afflictions involving Venus. Venus rules Taurus. Taurus is a fixed sign. Afflictions to the ruler of a sign cause afflictions in the sign or the mode, which in this case is fixed. The rules work. Venus afflicted can affect your heart as it rules a fixed sign. Venus afflicted also affects your circulation.

Jupiter rules the arteries or arterial circulation. The buildup of cholesterol or fat deposits in the arteries is a Jupiter Saturn or a Jupiter in Capricorn type of affliction. These are the things to look for in a chart for heart disease. If you are an asymptomatic type of person, look at your chart and see if you are prone to heart disease so you can work on preventive measures now. That is how medical astrology can help you.

We've discussed fixed signs in relation to heart disease. Jupiter in Leo or Aquarius or in the fifth or 11th houses (the fifth house is Leo; the 11th house is Aquarius – heart and circulation) with hard aspects from Saturn also being significators of coronary artery disease – CAD. Jupiter prominent and afflicted can cause problems. Jupiter used to rule Pisces before the discovery of Neptune. It has an involvement with the immune system. That's when Jupiter isn't so helpful, but I have seen it save people's lives activating the chart by transit or progression when they had a lot of very difficult health problems. Jupiter could augment a situation by making it worse or it can save your life. It depends on what else is going on in the chart.

Doane also gave another significator for arteriosclerosis. Coronary Artery Disease, the general term, is caused by arteriosclerosis or clogged arteries. She also cited Jupiter and the outer planets being prominent. There's Jupiter again because Jupiter rules arterial circulation and fat deposition in the body and too much fat can lead to hardening of the arteries. The liver can also be involved in that the liver produces the cholesterol that you don't get from food. There's Jupiter again which rules Sagittarius which rules the liver. The sign Virgo is also related anatomically to the liver.

Acute myocardial infarction (or a coronary thrombosis): the blood supply is cut off. Sun, Mars, Uranus with a connection to the fifth house or to Leo. There are other causes of sudden death besides the heart.

Audience: Are you saying that all three have to be in an aspect?

D.C.: Yes, you will most likely find Sun, Mars and Uranus connected in some way. One thing about a real life and death situation in medical astrology is that it won't be caused by one planet to one planet.

Another rule that works states that malefics afflicting angles or planets on angles indicate first-degree proneness to disease according to the mode. This is from *Essentials of Medical Astrology* by Dr. Harry Darling. Malefics (the outer planets and Mars) afflicting an angle, it doesn't matter what angle, or a malefic planet conjunct an angle, cause the greatest susceptibility to disease and the greatest life or death situation.

As an example, if you have Leo on an angle and natal Saturn is in hard aspect to that angle, it indicates a susceptibility to disease in the fixed cross since Leo is a fixed sign. Therefore, when you are analyzing a chart in terms of medical astrology if a person appears to have a really afflicted chart, but the planets are all in succedent houses, it is not as severe a problem. If there is a lot of activity involving the angles, which then get hit by transits or progressions, it is a more difficult situation. As Joanna Shannon used to say, you are looking for a "pileup," to describe a severe situation.

Sudden death could also result from drowning, an electrical shock or a stroke. Sudden death is a general term involving Sun, Mars, and Uranus. Uranus is sudden; the Sun is your body; Mars is the pain. Mars Uranus is pain and shock. Then add Leo or the fifth house for the heart.

Also Uranus in Taurus or Scorpio in hard aspect to the Sun or Moon. It could be a combination such as Sun or Moon in Scorpio, Sun or Moon in Taurus, Uranus in Taurus or Scorpio – some combination that makes a signature or what is called an astrological significator. Taurus rules the middle ear - which is a factor in dizziness.

Angina involves the fixed mode. This is from Charles Carter's book. His book is full of significators of diseases. He said heart disease can involve the Moon in Leo or Aquarius. And he found 24 degrees of Leo or Aquarius and 29 degrees of Gemini or Sagittarius to be involved in angina.

CARDIOMYOPATHIES

The next type of heart disease is cardiomyopathy which is an umbrella term for diseases of the heart muscle. This isn't a heart attack. Again the heart muscle is Leo and the circulation is Aquarius. Look for afflictions to the Sun, Leo or the fifth house. Understanding the heart from a medical perspective takes years to learn, but the astrology information seems to keep repeating itself. Malefics to the cusp of the fifth house or in opposition to it. Malefics in the fifth house or ruling it. Saturn in Leo making a difficult aspect to the Sun or Moon or Sun or Moon in Leo receiving a difficult aspect from Saturn. All of these could indicate diseases of the heart muscle. Saturn in Leo is called a lazy heart. As previously mentioned, wherever Saturn is in your chart, that organ ruled by the sign it is in gets the least blood supply. That part of the body needs to be nourished.

Therefore, Saturn in Leo can be a lazy heart and Saturn in Aquarius can indicate poor circulation. You need more oxygen or you need more exercise so the oxygen gets around. Always check the sign position of Saturn. It's very important.

Doane used 100 charts of heart disease and I believe she was talking about cardiomyopathies, which are diseases of the heart muscle. And she found that in 98% of the charts, Mars was prominent. In 96% of the charts the Sun was prominent and 93% Venus was prominent. Progressions – 100% of them had a progression of the Sun, 99% had a progression of Mars, 98% with Venus. Charts with one or more heavy discordant aspects – 100%.

She did not use the progressed Moon. The progressed Moon usually shows your emotional state during a particular month. You may not see disease with the progressed Moon but you could see less vitality such as the progressed Moon contacting Saturn.

INFECTION OF THE HEART VALVES

Besides cardiomyopathies which affect the heart muscle, there are also infections that attack the heart valves. For example, Rheumatic Heart Disease can cause the heart valves to be susceptible to a serious infection called bacterial endocarditis. Acute bacterial endocarditis usually attacks heart valves but occasionally can also attack other susceptible sites. Rheumatic Heart Disease is one of the contributing factors of this infection, because during the acute fever stage, the heart valves swell and thicken and later become a susceptible infection site. One of the most common causes of bacterial endocarditis is from dental work, which allows bacteria to get into the blood stream and latch on to a susceptible site that is usually a heart valve. IV drug abuse is another major cause of bacterial endocarditis. Astrologically, with infection you will see Neptune usually in combination with the Sun or Mars or Mars in Pisces. Also Mars Neptune combinations.

Doane did a study of Rheumatic Heart Disease and found Mars Saturn afflictions especially when they were afflicting each other. Mars is your fight and if Saturn is afflicting Mars, you don't have as much ability to fight.

LEO AND CANCER, MARS AND PLUTO

Pericarditis is an inflammation of the lining of the heart. Here is where the cardinal signs come in. The sign Cancer rules the linings of the body. The inner heart lining, the endocardium and the outer lining, the pericardium (the sac), are ruled by Cancer. So look for Cancer Leo combinations for more information on infectious diseases of the heart. I also think Pluto should be included as Pluto rules bacteria. If someone were suffering with bacterial endocarditis, they would have afflictions in Cancer and the involvement of Pluto or Mars. Pluto is a higher octave of Mars. Pluto can be tremendous infection and inflammation. And Mars can be less so. With both Mars and Pluto together you have a strong case for infection and inflammation.

CONGENITAL HEART DISEASE

Marcia Starck cites a 1977 study of congenital heart disease in her first book on medical astrology. Taurus was found to be the leader among sun signs with Aquarius and Leo following. Likewise succedent houses were also emphasized in the horoscope, and you will also find Saturn Venus afflictions.

Even though we don't understand all these types of heart diseases since we are not cardiologists, we understand fixed, and we see Leo and Aquarius showing up frequently, sometimes Cancer because it rules the lining of the heart.

There are diseases that can afflict any of the four heart valves, which include mitral valve disease, aortic valve disease, tricuspid valve disease and pulmonary valve disease. Any of these valves can leak, called insufficiency, or can become stenotic (calcified and thickened), or be attacked by a bacterial infection, (bacterial endocarditis). Neptune rules leakage; Saturn is thickening; Neptune and Pluto both could be involved in bacterial infection. This is the one type of heart disease that doesn't have a lot of astrological information. Darling gave Cancer as the ruler of the valves. When you look at Rex Bill's rulership book, he gives Uranus for the ruler of the valves. I feel it has to be Aquarius as Aquarius is co-ruled by Saturn and Uranus. The purpose of the valves is to move the blood forward and prevent backflow of blood in the heart. And therefore it seems like Aquarius which rules circulation makes more sense to rule the heart valves. And it goes along with the Leo Aquarius axis.

I think as astrologers all you have to recognize is heart disease. We are not going to be treating heart disease. So you can look at your own chart or maybe someone else's and mention that the chart shows a tendency toward heart disease and that they should have regular checkups and be on a heart-healthy diet. That's about as much as you can tell someone. This is information for you when you are advising clients unless you are also an M.D. Then you would have a greater understanding of the heart then we do as astrologers.

Other significators of the heart valves include: Uranus afflictions in Leo, Saturn affliction in Leo or the fifth house and Sun Saturn combinations.

Other forms of heart disease are associated with poor functioning of the endocrine glands, chronic lung diseases that overtax the heart, serious anemia, some nutritional diseases, poisoning from heavy metals or kidney waste such as uremia. So again, it's not always just the heart muscle and circulation.

URANUS: ARRHYTHMIAS, TACHYCARDIA & HEART MURMUR

Arrhythmias are functional disorders of the electrical system of the heart where the rhythm of the heart is interrupted. Arrhythmia is an umbrella term for many types of irregular heart rhythms and can include rapid and slow heartbeats, skipped beats and extra beats. A common arrhythmia is atrial fibrillation, which causes the atrium of the heart to "flutter," thus not allowing the ventricle to properly fill. This is usually not fatal, but if not treated with anticoagulants, the blood can pool in the atrium, thus causing clots. In most patients with atrial fibrillation, attempts are made to return the irregular rhythm back to normal. If medicine is unsuccessful, using a defibrillator, which shocks the heart can convert the arrhythmia.

Ventricular fibrillation similarly causes a "flutter" of the ventricle, which can be fatal. Even if the atrium "flutters", the ventricle can still fill. But if the ventricle "flutters", then little blood would circulate in the body, and death would be imminent. Ventricular fibrillation is usually the last stage the heart goes through before death. If a heart attack is followed by ventricular fibrillation, it's usually fatal.

Rapid heart rhythm is called tachycardia. This is where Uranus comes in since it rules the electrical system of the heart. And you will find with arrhythmia's that Uranus will be prominent. Uranus will be making an aspect to the Sun or the Moon; there will be an involvement of Leo or Aquarius. Marcia Starck found cases where the progressed fifth house cusp moved into the sixth house where they might have had Uranus and they developed an arrhythmia. You can watch your fifth house cusp by progression. Afflictions to Aquarius, Uranus fixed in Aquarius – all of these have to do with arrhythmia which is the function or the action of the heart.

A heart murmur is an abnormal heart sound that a physician hears with a stethoscope. A heart murmur could be Venus in a fixed sign afflicted by Uranus.

You might want to use midpoints such as the heart muscle: Sun/Mars or Sun/Jupiter.

So Saturn in Leo could indicate a weak or lazy heart that needs exercise and Saturn in Aquarius can be an indication of poor circulation.

Harmon found that 7 degrees of the mutables and 25 of the cardinals show up in heart disease.

CASES OF HEART DISEASE

Let's look at some charts of persons with heart disease. The first example is that of a male who had bypass surgery. He has the following significators for heart disease:

Mars conjunct Pluto in Leo; Mars ruling
5th house cusp
Saturn Uranus afflictions
Sun Saturn: cardiac disorder – the semi-sextile
can be considered a health aspect.
Sun conjunct Jupiter: heart disease
Mars in Leo: heart palpitation (perhaps brought
on by a thyroid problem), rheumatic heart disease,
angina pectoris

He is a fixed sign rising but there are no malefics affecting the Ascendant. Jupiter makes a sesquiquadrate to the Ascendant which brings in the involvement of the arteries.

Doris Chase Doane did longevity studies and found that people who live the longest have a good aspect between the Sun and Mars, or the Sun and Jupiter or Mars angular. So that's another thing you look for. You may have very difficult aspects in your chart, but if you have compensating aspects then even during difficult transits or progressions, you'll be able to fight disease. And you can also prevent disease by remaining non-toxic. Don't let the toxins build up in your body to begin with. If you see you are very sick, you may be retaining toxins and you could try to detoxify your body through nutritional measures. I wanted to mention using midpoints in analyzing heart disease. You can look at the Sun/Uranus midpoint which has to do with the pulse and breathing and possibly

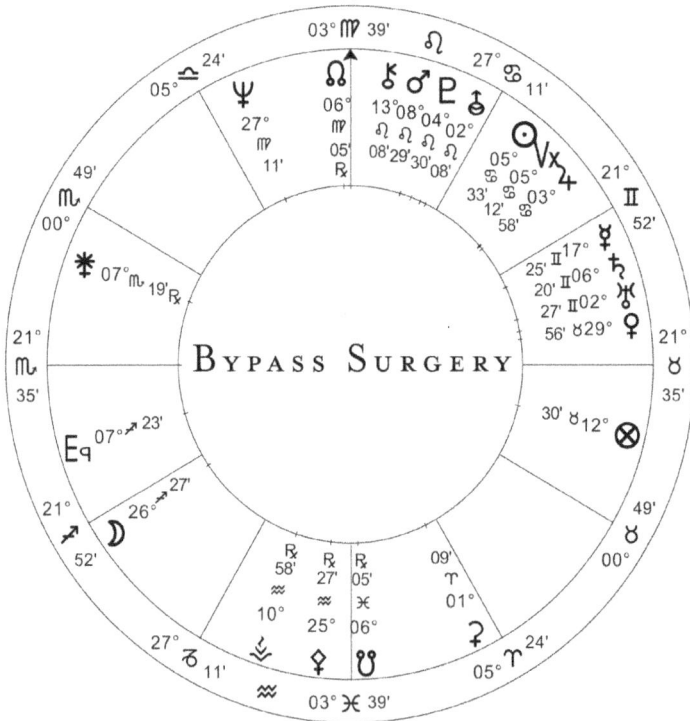

BYPASS SURGERY

problems with the heart. And Sun/Uranus can indicate heart neurosis.

You can look at the Moon/Uranus midpoint. It has to do with emotional tension and disturbances with blood pressure. You can check Mars/Jupiter – that's the heart muscle. You can check Saturn/Uranus. That could indicate a heart block or inhibitions of rhythm if configured with a personal point. And Uranus/Neptune can describe heart failure or paralysis of the rhythmic processes. Ebertin's book has a description of each midpoint in terms of the body. It's listed under Biological Correspondences. Most astrologers cite Ebertin when referring to midpoints.

In terms of midpoints for the Bypass Surgery chart his Sun = Mars/Uranus. Mars/Uranus can refer to surgery. Pluto = Sun/Uranus. MC = Saturn/Uranus.

We will look at the day of the bypass – Mar 29, 2000. Look at your eclipses before and after an event. They are energizers. On Jul 28, 1999 a lunar eclipse in 4 Aquarius 57 fell opposite his Mars Pluto conjunction in Leo. On January 21, 2000 a lunar eclipse in 00 Leo 26 fell conjunct natal Pluto. And on Feb 5, 2000 a solar eclipse in 16 Aquarius 01 was widely square his Ascendant. Transiting Mars was square natal Pluto in Leo the day of surgery. (Chapter Ten has more information on eclipses.)

The Darling book says that you can look back on various directions, progression, etc. and see when a condition may have begun. His progressed Sun had entered Virgo giving a potential concern with health.

In a worst case scenario when death is imminent, you can look at the chart and find several difficult combinations hitting at once. Also, remember this. You've lived through lots of difficult transits and progressions without getting sick. Sometimes it's psychological changes or events; the roof will fall in but you're healthy. I don't believe in predicting illness. Just look at the transits and progressions, etc. when you develop a condition to see how long it might last. I would never predict illness for someone and say you will get this or that. I give a general reading and talk about what's coming up, but you can talk about health issues in terms of periods of stress and less vitality or resistance.

The next case Valve Replacement is that of a male who had four open-heart surgeries to replace heart valves. We will look at his chart in terms of significators for heart disease.

AFFLICTIONS TO THE SUN

Afflictions to the fifth house cusp or ruler of the fifth – Mars is opposite the fifth house cusp as well as conjunct the 11th house cusp; Mars is also in detriment.

> **Sun square Uranus:** ventricular fibrillation
> Afflictions in Cancer or cardinal signs: affecting lining of the heart
> Sun Uranus: arterial fibrillation, ventricular fibrillation
> Mars in Taurus: affects middle ear – dizziness – leading to blockage of blood vessels and coronary thrombosis
> Mars sesquiquadrate Saturn: heart block
> Neptune in Leo: weak heart, low blood pressure from sluggish activity of the heart

Uranus = Mars/Saturn. Uranus is elevated in the chart and is associated with the action of the heart valves. Earlier I mentioned the Saturn/Uranus midpoint can indicate a heart block or inhibitions of rhythm if configured with a personal point. His MC = Saturn/Uranus by semisquare. Pluto is conjunct and parallel the Ascendant which can indicate bodily transformation. The sign position of

25° ♓ 56'

02° ♉ 01'

27° ♒ 41'

14°07' ♈ ♈
53'17'

17° ♓ 10'

00°
09° ♉ ♉
04°
06° 13° 02'

30'
11° Ⅱ

♊ ♌ 09° Ⅱ
18'

15° ♒

♀ 05° ♒ 22'

♀ 14° R

♀ 26° Ⅱ 35'
♀ 03° ♋ 06'
☉ 04° ♋ 32'
☿ 09° ♋ 21' R
♇ 16° ♋ 20'
☊ 25° ♋ 47'

15° ♋ 49'

VALVE

REPLACEMENT

SURGERY

15° ♑ 49'

05° ♌ 22'

02° ♌
27° ♍

55' ♍ 12'

06' ♏
24' ♏ 21° ♎ 02°

R 25' ♐
18' 23' 14°
09° ♐
02° ♄

30'
11° ♐ ☋ Vx

Ψ

✳ ☾

27° ♌ 41'

25° ♍ 56' ♎

02° ♏ 01'

Neptune can indicate a lack of tone in that area. Even though it appears to affect an entire generation, when included as part of a group of significators, it adds to the indications.

Former Vice-President Dick Cheney has a history of heart problems going back to 1978. He has the following significators for heart disease.

Afflictions to the Sun as well as a planet in Leo
Pluto quincunx his 5th house cusp
A malefic in the eleventh houses
Afflictions to planets in Aquarius

Jupiter Saturn (cholesterol deposits). Jupiter is both conjunct and parallel Saturn.
Mars quincunx Uranus
Sun square Saturn: cardiac disorder
Sun sesquiquadrate Neptune – weak heart
Fixed emphasis – rigidity and faulty elimination causing toxins in blood
Sun square Jupiter – potential for heart disease

Uranus is elevated in his chart and is contraparallel to his Sun in Aquarius. Sun Uranus is associated with ventricular fibrillation.

On June 30, 2001 Cheney had a pacemaker implanted to help normalize his heart rhythms. Transiting Neptune was applying to his natal Sun indicating further heart problems and closely square his Jupiter Saturn conjunction in Taurus. On that day Uranus in Aquarius was conjunct Mercury in Aquarius. Transiting Mars was also conjunct natal Mars. Cheney experienced other episodes of heart disease at other times in his life such as a blocked artery that could be signified by his Jupiter Saturn conjunction. He has had three heart attacks along with episodes of ir-regular heart rhythm. All can be seen in his natal chart. .

Audience: Would an opposition of the Sun and Uranus be as detrimental to the heart if they were in other signs than Leo and Aquarius?

DC: I think it's stronger for heart disease when it is in Leo and Aquarius, but any hard aspect to the Sun can indicate weakened heart action. That is because the Sun rules Leo, which is the heart muscle. Leo Aquarius is the heart axis but you can have other indications in the chart that lessen the severity. You need to study the chart and see how many significators there are for heart disease.

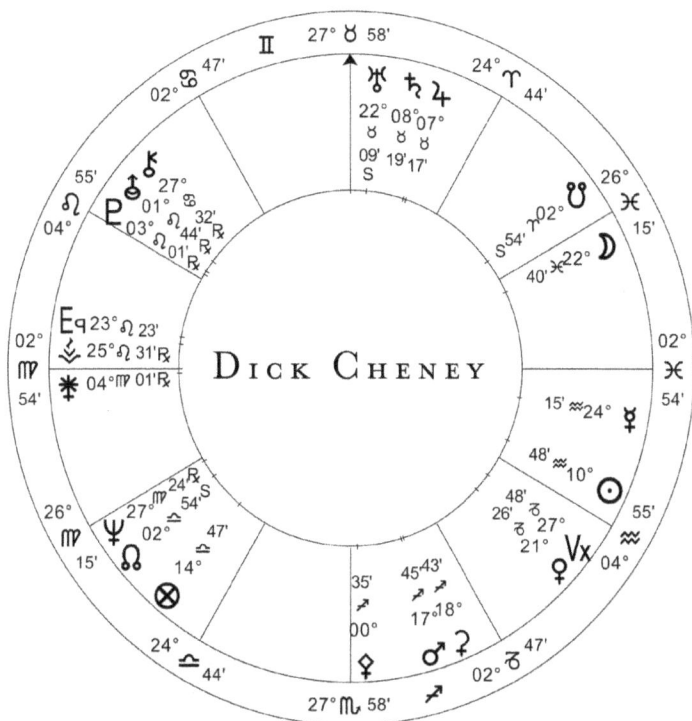

Audience: Can you recommend any other books?

DC: *Mind and Body in Astrology* is good. The Nauman book can be used like a textbook. In order to understand medical astrology, you have to learn about anatomy and physiology. The Davidson book is a good introduction. The Darling book is also very good. For predictions you can use the Davison book which has some medical information in it. The Carter book is just a good book to have. The Marcia Starck books are also excellent introductions to medical astrology. My newest book *Managing Your Health and Wellness* can be used as a textbook for medical astrology.

How to Give an Astrological Health Reading has a chapter on Heart Disease.

1. Bills, Rex E.: *The Rulership Book,* Macoy Publishing & Masonic Supply Co., Inc., Richmond, Virginia, 1976

2. Carter, C.E.O.: *An Encyclopaedia Of Psychological Astrology,* The Theosophical Publishing House Ltd., London, England, 1963

3. Cramer, Diane: *How To Give An Astrological Health Reading,* AFA, Tempe, AZ, 1996.

4. Cramer, Diane: *Managing Your Health and Wellness,* Llewellyn Publications, Woodbury, MN, 2006.

5. Darling, Harry F.: *Essentials Of Medical Astrology,* American Federation of Astrologers, Inc., Tempe, Arizona, 1981

6. Davidson, William: *Davidson's Medical Astrology,* Astrological Bureau, Monroe, New York, 1979

7. Davison, R.C., *The Technique of Prediction,* L.N. Fowler & Col. Ltd., London, England, 1972.

8. Doane, Doris Chase: *Astrology 30 Years Research,* American Federation of Astrologers, Inc., Tempe, Arizona, 1979

9. Ebertin, Reinhold: *Combination of Stellar Influences.* Evertin-Verlag, Aalen, Germany, 1972.

10. Harmon, J. Merrill: *Complete Astro-Medical Index,* Astro- Analytics Publications, Van Nuys, California, 1979.

11. Harvey, Ronald: *Mind & Body In Astrology,* L.N. Fowler & Co., Ltd., Essex, England, 1983.

12. Nauman, Eileen: *The American Book Of Nutrition & Medical Astrology,* Astro Computing Services, San Diego, CA, 1982.

13. Starck, Marcia: *Astrology Key To Holistic Health.* Seek-It Publications, Birmingham, Michigan, 1982.

14. Starck, Marcia: *Medical Astrology, Healing for the 21st Century,* Earth Medicine Books, Santa Fe, NM, 2002.

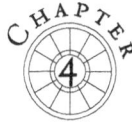

MENTAL ABERRATIONS
IN THE CHART

In this chapter you will learn how to recognize mental disorders in the natal chart through the use of astrological significators and chart examples. You will find a summary of major astrological configurations involved in mental disorders as well as the use of midpoints and planets in declination. A bibliography of astrology books that contain information on mental disorders will aid you in further research.

I'm going to define what I think of as a mental aberration. Anything that keeps you from performing or working or enjoying your life is a mental aberration. That's my own definition, which is why you see the charts of Dick Cavett and Mike Wallace. Both experienced tremendous depression that was debilitating to them. So in my opinion mental aberration is something that debilitates you, be it depression or schizophrenia; they're all still problems. There are nine charts that I will use to point out various mental disorders. Some of the charts were given to me by colleagues who knew these people. One chart, the multiple personality example, came from Lois Rodden's database.

And then I chose some celebrities because it's fun to see what's going on in their lives. So what did I learn?

When you're doing a health reading and you're looking to see if someone has heart disease or a stomach problem, it's pretty obvious. It's not obvious when you're a beginner. I'll say that about astrology. It's pretty obvious if you know what you're doing and you know your significators. Mental problems are the least obvious of them all because it might just be a personality quirk that you're looking at or you could be schizoid without being schizophrenic. So you're not going to see mental problems necessarily by looking at a chart and saying, "Wow, this person is manic depressive; this person is schizophrenic." When we go through the schizophrenic's chart, as you go into the chart, you pull out the information.

You must use midpoints in my opinion. If you're a beginner it may be too difficult for you. It's the study of Cosmobiology and you use the Combination of Stellar Influences by Ebertin[7] and you just look up the meaning of the midpoints. You also need to use parallels of declination because someone might have a Sun Uranus parallel for example, but not have that aspect in longitude in the natal chart. And that may show some quirkiness. You do need to look at parallels of declination.

As I've mentioned, I also use the 22½ degree aspect. I have the Janus program and it's easy for me to show the 22½ degree aspect which is half of a semi-square. If you keep it close to exact, not more than 30" of orb, you'll be surprised at what you'll see as far as it being a hard aspect. I'm still an old-fashioned astrologer who thinks there are hard and soft aspects. So a 22½ is a hard aspect. And I found that aspect will also give you information.

This was a fairly new topic for me. So we'll review what other astrologers wrote about mental illness or mental aberrations and then we'll go through the charts examples.

So what kinds of indications do you look for? By the way you can look for specific significators of a problem and not see the condition. The condition can be seen by something else such as a singleton or an unaspected planet or something that stands out in the chart that makes that person different.

Jane Ridder Patrick[10] says that mutability has a lot to do with mental diseases or what she calls "diseases of distraction." So sometimes a lot of mutability can indicate nervousness or mental disorders. Never make assumptions on any of this information. You know when you practice astrology you're looking for a lot of indications in the chart. One indication is not enough.

Mutability can describe diseases of distraction, irrational behavior, nervousness, irritability. Too much excessive mental activity, according to Jane Patrick Ridder, means you're out of touch with the reality of a situation and you're very busy; you don't think there's enough time to do everything; you make yourself a nervous wreck. Or you just suffer with irrational fears. And the main thing she says is to learn to focus your attention. This will help you get rid of a lot of this nervousness or irrationality. Sometimes when you're looking at a chart with many difficult aspects and there's a lot of mutability, the excess mutability can be an added mental component of the chart.

Now Cornell[4] in the *Encyclopaedia of Medical Astrology* gives the following for abnormal and mental trouble. And sometimes you'll see this and sometimes you won't: Neptune afflicted in the 3rd or 9th house. Obviously, if it's the 3rd or 9th, these are mental houses. So afflictions involving the 3rd or 9th houses can sometimes produce mental problems. And some astrologers say especially if there's a water sign involved. There seems to be a greater tendency to mental problems when there's a lot of water in the chart. Now he (Cornell) also mentioned Neptune afflicted in the 3rd or 9th especially if there is also a square or opposition to Saturn or Mars in the chart. So if Neptune has some connection with the 3rd or 9th house, and this could include hard aspects from Neptune to third or ninth house planets and Mars or Saturn is also involved, this could indicate mental troubles.

A.T. Mann[9] has a book on medical astrology. He states that birth traumas are responsible for many types of illnesses, both psychological and physical. The primary reason he feels is that in the last century the rising increase in the power of the medical profession has transformed childbirth from a natural process to a pathological medical procedure. He feels the dehumanization of birth is seen by many to be the primary factor in the difficulties of our modern society – that your individual birth process sets you off for the rest of your life, psychologically or physi- cally. You can't tell all the time when you're looking at a chart if you're being affected psychologically or physically. A.T. Mann feels that the birth process can affect you psychologically. He uses the aspects to the Ascendant to describe what was going on around you during the birth process. For example Mars could be some kind of a violent influence such as damage from the use of forceps and Saturn could be repressive and therefore the whole birth process affects you psychologically.

Reinhold Ebertin[6] talks about combinations involving Neptune and Pluto. This could be in a midpoint; it could be connected to personal points. He associates Neptune and Pluto with confusion, hysteria and the ill effects of toxic stimulants including tobacco. Sometimes a mental disorder is caused by someone taking the wrong drug, for example. There can be psychological symptoms followed by functional disorders. And then he talks about Uranus and Neptune that gives you the ability to switch off the conscious mind and turn yourself over to the uncontrolled impulses of the unconscious mind. So you can lose it, in other words, if you've got some hard aspects connected with Uranus and Neptune.

Ronald Harvey[8] has some interesting concepts in his book on medical astrology. He separates manic depression from schizophrenia. First he talks about a combination of fire and water in the chart for manic depression. He says fire and water suggest an instinctive impulsive tendency if instability is indicated. The important thing is to first see if instability is indicated in the chart. Then if other indications show up, you might conclude that the chart shows a tendency toward a mental disorder. Otherwise, it can be instability without being manic depression or schizophrenia. Or it's someone who is moody. There's a fine line between somebody who's a little quirky to being a schizophrenic when examining a chart. I think you'll see that once we do the sample charts, that the schizophrenics do have very difficult charts.

Harvey says if instability is indicated, there can be an inclination to swing from one pole to the other, from impulsiveness (fire) to withdrawal (water), from rashness (fire) to timidity (water), from self-expression to self-destruction and back again. And the tendency to push too far describes a manic depressive.

Then he talks about air and earth for schizophrenia. Again, this would be if other indications show up in the chart. There is a tendency to deliberate, logical decisions and actions with air and earth. Here he finds the person is more cool and critical with less of an emotional swing. If instability is indicated in the chart, this type is more prone to nervous behavior and oscillation rather than emotional swings, which is the fire-water combination. This air-earth combination could be schizophrenic if pushed to extremes.

Harvey states that with manic depressives, you're going to have a Jupiterian influence. You know those highs and lows of Jupiter. He claims a combination of Jupiter with Uranus and Pluto or Jupiter with Neptune can cause those highs and lows that have to do with manic depression, especially Jupiter and Neptune. Sometimes you'll see a Jupiter Neptune combination in a schizophrenic's chart. This is what I mean when I said you have to take all the significators, and they will sometimes work and sometimes not work. You will see this as we go through the charts. It can be harder to see exactly the type of mental aberration.

Then Harvey talks about the schizophrenic type of personality being more brittle, jagged and nervous. So this would be Saturn with Uranus or Neptune. So the Jupiter would be more manic depressive and the Saturn, Uranus and Neptune along with air and earth would be more of a schizophrenic type.

Audience: Air and earth?

DC: Yes, air and earth for schizophrenia and fire and water for manic depression. And he says for any tendency toward abnormality you have to look at the outer planets, Uranus, Neptune and Pluto with the Sun, Moon, Mercury or Ascendant/Descendant. In other words if you're looking for abnormalities, it will have something to do with Uranus, Neptune or Pluto and a personal point. And especially if Mercury is involved. And you would think the first thing I would have said to you is that Mercury causes mental illness. Yes, but you could have an afflicted Mercury and also have nervous diseases or respiratory disorders. You can't always tell; that's the thing. Certainly Mercury is the planet of the mind and you want to look at it for mental disorders. Mental disorders involve a combination of indicators which is why we're going to start with some of the charts so you can see what I'm trying to describe and then we'll continue on with more significators.

I wanted to mention to you to use the Merck Manual[1] (they now have a home edition). It has very good definitions of all diseases. And what I find helpful is that you can take a definition of a particular disorder and then figure out what planets or combination of planets describe the disorder and look for them in the chart. It's a good way to learn medical astrology.

SCHIZOPHRENIA

We're going to start with the two schizophrenic charts. Schizophrenia is defined as a serious mental disorder characterized by lack of contact with reality. The person suffers with psychosis, hallucinations, delusion, false beliefs, abnormal thinking, disruptive work and social functioning. According to the Merck Manual schizophrenia affects under 1% of the population, but ¼ of all hospital beds in this country are occupied by schizophrenics. And 20% of social security disability goes to schizophrenics. So it's quite a problem and it may have to do with genetic predisposition of a problem that occurs before, during or after birth or as a result of a violent infection of the brain. Medical experts really don't know the exact cause of these mental disorders.

Look at the first chart – Schizophrenia & Paranoia (female), the 12 Leo rising chart. Now I always felt paranoia had to do with Mercury Pluto combinations. When you look at this chart there is no Mercury Pluto aspect in longitude, but there is a contra-parallel of Mercury to Pluto. So be sure to check your parallels and contra-parallels.

Also, look at that difficult T-square on the angles. We have Uranus rising opposite the Sun square Neptune. There's your Sun, Uranus, Neptune – a very difficult combination especially on an angle. Sun Uranus can indicate states of tension and a contradictory nature. Sun Neptune can indicate chaotic conditions. Ebertin says that Uranus Neptune can describe losing control of the waking consciousness which leads to a lack of clearness, instability, lack of emotional balance and a confused psychic state. There is a Moon Neptune aspect by 22½ degrees that I wouldn't even know if I hadn't set my computer to see the 22½ degree aspects, and there's also a Jupiter Neptune 22½ degree aspect. Moon Neptune and Jupiter Neptune can indicate poor judgment. Moon is semi-square Pluto. It's pretty wide and normally I wouldn't use a semi- square at 3 degrees orb but A.T. Mann says that Moon Pluto is a significator of schizophrenia.

We've got Uranus on the Ascendant, which adds to an erratic personality. Neptune is square the Ascendant, which can describe someone who is confused, disoriented and moody. Not everyone who has these aspects acts like this so there's probably something genetic that we don't know about along with the astrological significators.

Here are some midpoint interpretations in the chart taken from the *Combination of Stellar Influences.*[4]

Moon = Mercury/Saturn
a retarded development of mind and soul.

Mars = Moon/Saturn
self critical to the point of torment, soul conflicts.

Mars = Uranus/Pluto
a violent state of precipitation.

Saturn = Mars/Ascendant
inability to develop and express one's potential in the right way.

Saturn = Sun/Jupiter
incompatibility, inhibitions partly caused organically.

Uranus = Mars/MC
the inclination to become furious or violent. There's the MC thrown into it so we have a personal point.

Uranus = Mars/Neptune
states of weakness emerging suddenly.

Neptune = Moon/Mars
a misdirected emotional life.

Pluto = Saturn/Neptune
emotional depression, a serious illness.

Ascendant = Moon/Uranus
easily excitable.

Right there we have some very difficult midpoints. When I see one of those midpoints in a chart I don't get that carried away. When I see several of them, you have to figure there's something not right here. And then you look at that T-square. What's the planet elevated in the chart – Mars – proneness to violence, irritability and impatience.

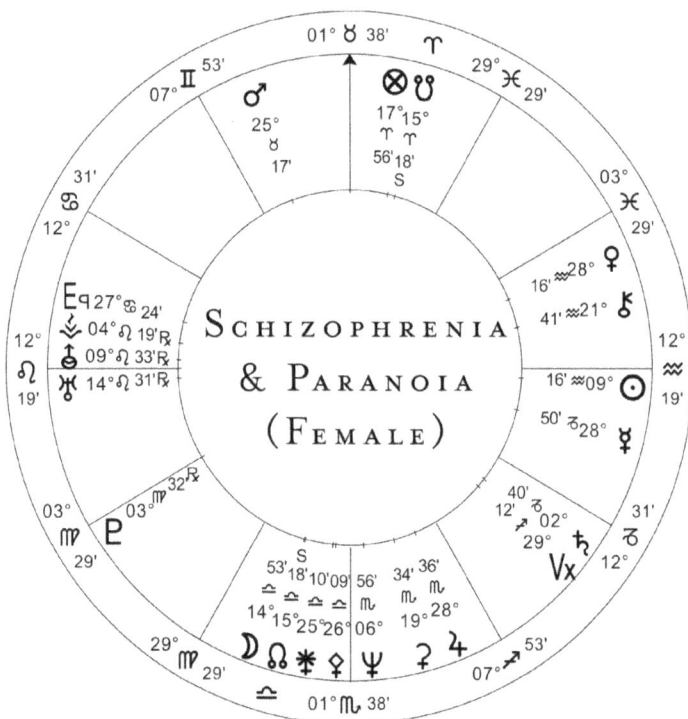

SCHIZOPHRENIA & PARANOIA (FEMALE)

What really made me look at these charts and go "wow" was when I looked at the next chart called Schizophrenia (Male), and I also saw a similar pattern. The first example had Sun Uranus Neptune. Schizophrenia (male) also has Sun square Uranus and Neptune is conjunct the Sun. That's the same three planets. I only used two schizophrenic charts and after studying the charts for a while I noticed the similarities between the two charts. The Sun Neptune conjunction would be considered out of sign. This is called a dissociate aspect. According to **Skyscript. co.uk**: "Dissociate aspects are considered weakened in

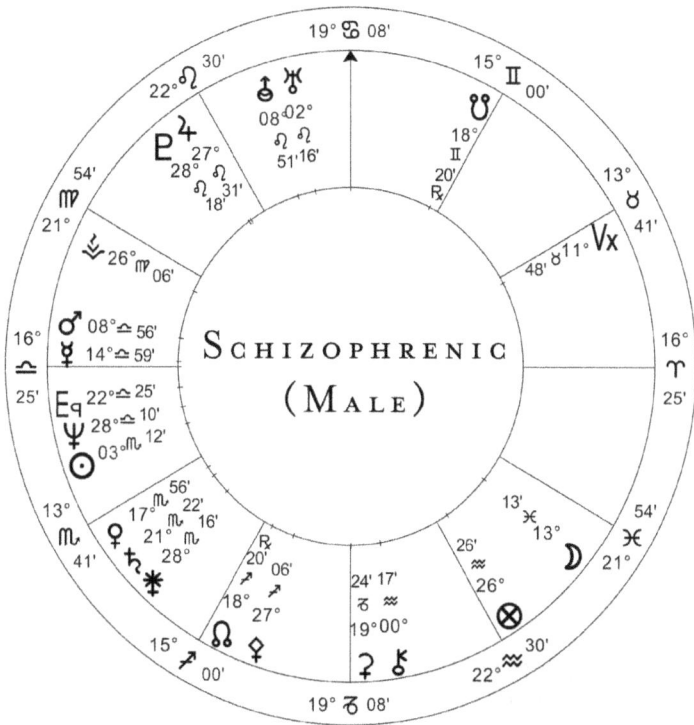

SCHIZOPHRENIC
(MALE)

effect, or represent a contradictory principle or barrier which needs to be overcome in order for the aspect to fully express itself." In my opinion this intensifies the difficulty of this conjunction.

Both charts have an emphasis in fixed signs, a lot of rigidity. The second one has Mars conjunct the Ascendant. It's pretty wide. There's a Mercury Mars conjunction to the Ascendant and it could describe the way schizophrenia's scream a lot, the ones I've noticed anyway. Or maybe it's a lack of awareness of what they're saying – Mercury Mars conjunction in the subconscious 12th house also conjunct the Ascendant.

MIDPOINTS:

Sun = Mercury/Saturn
a person with a retarded mental development.

Sun = Saturn/Ascendant
difficult circumstances of life.

Mars = Jupiter/Saturn
a lack of endurance or tenaciousness, discontent, an inconstant will.

Mars = Saturn/Pluto
brutality, violence, having to fight for one's existence.

Mars = Uranus/Nodes
the tendency to get excited easily in the presence of others, quarrelling, exercising self-control only with the greatest difficulty.

Uranus = Mercury/Saturn
great inner tension, excitability, incompatibility, a disease of the nerves.

Uranus = Saturn/Neptune
self-willed, obstinate.

Neptune = Mars/Saturn
insufficient power to tackle things.

Ascendant = Moon/Saturn
inhibition of development.

Again, with this second example it was the midpoints that stood out. And another thing I noticed was that there were no planets in earth in schizophrenia (Male). What do you think that means? Out of touch with reality? They say when you have a lack of earth you're not grounded which is why it's helpful to eat heavy foods to ground you. If you put all this together and you have no earth, too much rigidity – the fixed emphasis and the combination of the Sun, Uranus and Neptune – out of touch with reality plus you add all these midpoints, you've got a person who might have a mental disorder. Notice the planets all around the Ascendant. And what's elevated in this chart – Uranus. In the other chart Mars was elevated. Elevated planets have a lot to do with describing your personality. They're not, in my opinion, necessarily so much having to do with the profession as much as a psychological indicator of what you're looking for in life or a mode of behavior. Always look for the planet closest to the MC even if it's not that close. It's still the most elevated planet in the chart if there's nothing else in that hemisphere. And it tells a lot about what you're like. Any questions about the schizophrenics?

Audience: How does Pluto affect when it's in a midpoint?

DC: With a midpoint you're using three factors. So it's just one more factor. With Pluto you've got extremes. And/or there's an obsessive quality about Pluto or Scorpio or something you can't let go of.

Here's a definition of manic depression from the Merck Manual.[1] It is also called bi-polar disorder, a condition in which periods of depression alternate with periods of mania or lesser degrees of excitement. It affects slightly less than 2% of the population, is believed to be hereditary and usually begins in the teens, twenties, or thirties.

Depression is described as a feeling of intense sadness out of proportion to the extent of an event, and it persists beyond an appropriate period of time. So it's out of proportion to the event, and it goes on too long. 10% of people who see a doctor for a physical problem are also depressed. When we get to it, the multiple personality disorder example, the new name is – associative identity disorder. There's no such thing anymore as a multiple personality – it's an associative identity disorder. That would be the chart labeled Multiple Personality. It is a condition in which two or more identities or personalities alternate and control a person's behavior in which there are episodes of amnesia; they are more likely to commit suicide than people with any other mental disorder. It is found in three to four percent of people hospitalized for other psychiatric problems. Most of them – 97 - 98% of them with associative identity disorder have suffered child abuse. So what would you look for in a chart? You would look for indications of child abuse as well as the indications of a mental disorder if you're looking for multiple personalities. Just briefly and I'll get to it, but the main thing that stood out for me in the chart of the multiple personality was that Neptune was rising. Otherwise I didn't think the condition was that obvious.

Here are more significators of depression.

Cornell[4]: What he says about depression and a lot of astrologers say this is that it's a Saturn disease. When you're looking for depression you're looking for Capricorn or Saturn in some way or planets in Capricorn or something associated with Saturn, which makes sense. And what's the standard aspect – Moon Saturn and probably secondarily Mercury Saturn for depression. Every astrology textbook you read that talks about depression mentions Moon Saturn. Saturn involved with Mercury and the Moon, Cornell says. He also says that Saturn Retrograde or Stationery could indicate depression. And that Saturn in the first, third or sixth house and in hard aspect or afflicted could have to do with depression. I certainly think Saturn in the third could since the third is a mental house. And he also says Saturn afflicted in Virgo could have to do with depression. And a Moon Neptune aspect could also have to do with depression.

Audience: What about signs?

DC: A lot of astrology books say water signs have to do with depression.

Melancholy and discontent. This is from Charles Carter.[3] Moon or Venus afflicted by Saturn or in Saturnine signs – so Moon in Capricorn, Venus in Capricorn or Moon or Venus to Saturn could be depression or melancholy. Especially if the third house is involved. Charles Carter says Venus afflicted by Mars destroys content and real happiness. He states that Venus square Saturn often gives a life of regret and sorrow unless other influences are powerfully contradicted. This was written at the beginning of the last century when astrologers were much more negative. You know anyone who has these aspects in their chart can go through some difficult times. So I wouldn't underestimate Venus Saturn or Moon Saturn. The watery signs also tend to moodiness. The fiery signs especially Sagittarius are either up or down. Libra, he states, is easily ruffled but soon recovers. And the air signs and Virgo have an intellectual placidity. So they're placid. Earth signs are usually content except Capricorn, which is easily depressed by snubs or slights.

More from Charles Carter: Pessimism as a general attitude is the result of heavy Saturn afflictions and weak benefic influences. If the ninth is involved, the attitude may take the form of a philosophy of life. The mutable signs, especially Virgo, experience the most with pessimism while the cardinal signs are far less liable to contract it. Apparently, if you have a lot of cardinality you shouldn't get too depressed. You're probably too busy. Who's got time? Carter says you have to examine the cadent houses because those are considered mental houses.

MORE SIGNIFICATORS

Gemini and Sagittarius can show up with manic depressives. Manic depressive is bi-polar. A Gemini - Sagittarius element involved, Neptune in the first. And sometimes Mars in the first or a poorly aspected Mars indicates a head injury which leads to the bi-polar disorder. Sometimes the disorder is literally caused by an accident to the head. Injury or accident at birth, birth trauma, whatever, can have to do with bi-polar disorders. Similarly, an emphasis in Gemini or Sagittarius could indicate the bi-polar condition.

I also have more information on midpoints that I can give you as significators.

Depression: Pluto = Moon/Saturn.

Emotional illness: Sun = Saturn/Neptune or Saturn = Pluto/Ascendant.

Schizophrenia could be Moon Pluto or Moon Uranus aspects. Many people have these aspects, so you can't make the assumption that if you have these aspects you are schizophrenic as you know that's not true.

Mental suffering: MC = Saturn/Neptune.

Depressive psychosis: Mercury = Neptune/MC.

Moodiness: Sun = Jupiter/Saturn.

I find Jupiter Saturn combinations show up a lot as inconstancy. One minute you're one way and another minute your mood changes. Another one for moodiness: Uranus = Moon/Neptune. The Moon rising is also associated with moodiness. In most cases these aspects will just signify moodiness or inconstancy and nothing more.

Violent insanity: Uranus = Mercury/Mars.

Anxiety: Moon Mars involved and the signs Cancer and Virgo involved. This is A.T. Mann.[9] And he also says that Mercury Uranus is nervous irritability. And Mercury Neptune describes anxiety states. And Moon Saturn can be neurosis, depressive psychosis, and Moon Saturn is another combination for anxiety.

Let's look at the charts of Dick Cavett and Mike Wallace for depression.

Mike Wallace lectures and so does Dick Cavett on depression and they have discussed the topic frequently, so I thought we should look at their charts. I said at the beginning that this information is not just about aberrations like schizophrenia, but it's anything that keeps you from having a happy life. We have Howard Hughes for paranoia. I thought it would be interesting to look at his chart.

Mike Wallace has Moon square Saturn and he also has Saturn conjunct Neptune. Saturn Neptune is another combination that keeps coming up as an indication of depression.

Let's look at Dick Cavett's chart.

We just said that Mike Wallace has a Saturn Neptune aspect. So does Dick Cavett. He has the opposition. He also is weak in the fire element. Weak fire in a chart can indicate low self-esteem. Aside from the medical issues such as poor digestion and low vitality for low fire, it also can indicate a lack of self esteem. So Dick Cavett, despite

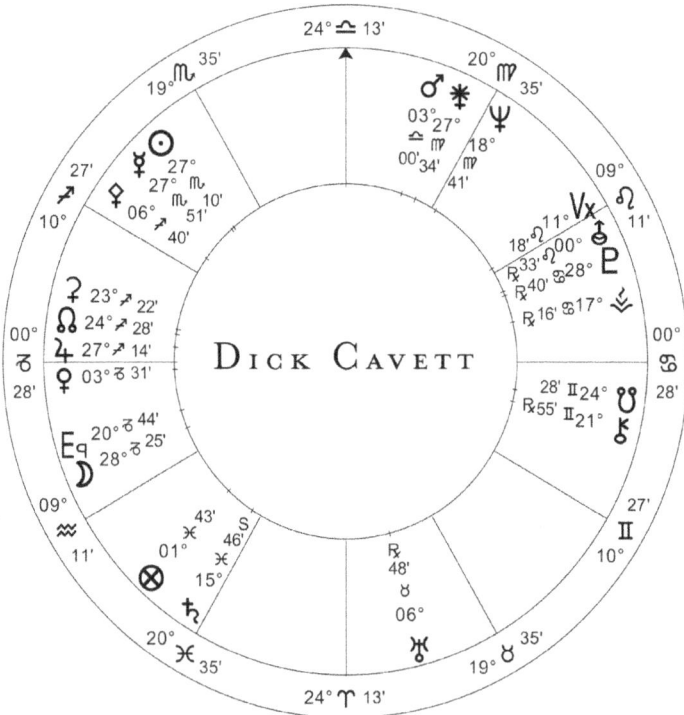

DICK CAVETT

his success, has low fire that may have contributed to his depression. He also has Neptune conjunct the ninth house. So there's that 9th house influence, and it rules his third house. So we've got that 3rd and 9th house component for mental problems or depression. He has Jupiter = Mars/Neptune – unhappiness or ill luck in the midst of wealth. That midpoint is also in the chart of Christopher Reeves, which I always thought was interesting. Dick Cavett has:

Venus = Saturn/Neptune
bad feelings.

Mars = Saturn/MC
feeling defenseless.

Saturn = Sun/Ascendant
inhibition and shyness.

Neptune = Uranus/Pluto
neuroses.

MC = Sun/Neptune
a negative outlook, periods of depression, hypersensitivity or mental or emotional stress.

Cavett has planets in Saturnine signs. He seems to be fitting the rules. Notice Venus rising in Capricorn and Capricorn rising. We've got the Saturnine signs. He's got Venus square Mars. Remember Carter said it shows a discontent with life. He has water signs which tend to moodiness. He's got a water sign on the third house cusp – Pisces. And then I looked up Saturn in Pisces. According to Sakonian.[11] *(The Astrologer's Handbook)*, Saturn afflicted in Pisces can indicate paranoia, extreme worry, fretfulness, regret over past mistakes and misfortune, which if carried too far will result in neurotic tendencies especially if Virgo is involved in some way. And here you have Saturn opposite Neptune in Virgo. Saturn opposite Neptune – a struggle between fantasy and reason. By the way, paranoids in general tend to blame everyone for their problems, and I was always taught that oppositions have to do with other people. So I would look for a lot of oppositions in a chart for paranoia, (see Howard Hughes) as someone who has a lot of oppositions could have paranoia or they blame. They don't see themselves realistically; it's the other person's fault.

So we've got that struggle between fantasy and reason and Cavett also has Moon semisquare Saturn. I'll accept it since it's just a little over 2 degrees. Cavett has the significators and also he has Moon in Capricorn opposite Pluto. He has those extremes. Here's a chart with all the significators of depression. The Saturnine signs, the Saturn Neptune, the Venus Mars, plus the midpoints I mentioned.

Now let's look some more at Mike Wallace's chart. Wallace has the Moon conjunct Mercury square Saturn conjunct Neptune. And it's pretty close and that is one of the prime indicators of depression and Moon Neptune is also anxiety. He also has Saturn parallel Pluto, which is a tough combination. Life can seem like a struggle at times. The Moon Mercury conjunction is in 00 degrees, a critical degree, which can add to the intensity of the combination.

MIDPOINTS FOR MIKE WALLACE INCLUDE:

Saturn = Sun/Mercury
a pessimistic attitude to life, a serious outlook on life.

Saturn = Sun/Moon
the state of feeling depressed.

MC = Sun/Neptune
a negative outlook.

Water signs tend to moodiness. He has Pisces rising. He has all mutable angles. What did we say at the beginning of the chapter? Mutability can have a mental component. I think Dick Cavett has a lot of mental significators for depression. Mike Wallace does with that Moon Mercury square Saturn Neptune. It's very strong. Dick Cavett is a textbook example.

Audience: What about Saturn?

DC: Saturn equals the Sun/Moon midpoint in Mike Wallace's chart by square. It is an indirect midpoint which some astrologers don't think is as strong as a direct midpoint. You know when you're doing midpoints you're doing an aspect to a midpoint which is indirect when it's a square, semi-square or sesquiquadrate and direct when it's a conjunction or opposition. All these years that I've been doing astrology, if you find a lot of significators, then it adds up.

Audience: Question on midpoints.

DC: Some of the midpoints I gave you were from A.T. Mann and some of them were from Ebertin. I kept switching between books. A.T. Mann[9] has a lot of significators at the end of his book *(Astrology and the Art of Healing)* on different diseases. Ebertin's books are out there – *Astrological Healing. The History and Practice of Astromedicine.*[6] And *The Combination of Stellar Influences*[7] is the main midpoint book.

Audience: What about the first house? (Dick Cavett)

DC: Yes, the first house with the Capricorn influence and also 00 degrees Capricorn Ascendant which is a critical degree. This makes it more intense. Of course 00 Capricorn is equal to the Aries point which is the world axis and that could be an indication of fame in Dick Cavett's chart.

Let's look at the two manic depressive charts. First is Manic Depressive Alcoholic (F). Do you notice there's a Mars Uranus opposition here? It's wide – 6 degrees but it's angular. I once read in William Davidson[5] *(Davidson's Medical Astrology)* that alcoholics drink due to a spasm condition in their body – to overcome the spasm. And this is the chart of somebody who has a Mars Uranus opposition. And Davidson said that Mars Uranus types could become alcoholics.

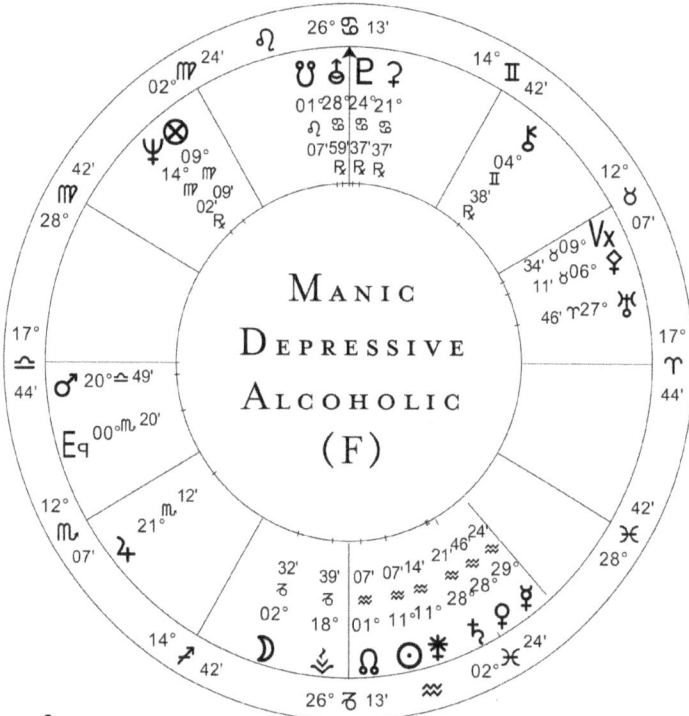

This manic depressive has a lot of air, so there's probably an overactive mind. Jupiter is square Saturn – inconstancy. Depression – the Moon is in Capricorn. We've got the highs and the lows. And look at that – you've got a stellium in Aquarius which could describe somebody very high strung or quirky. You've got Mercury conjunct Saturn with Venus thrown in so you could see this as highs and lows also. The Sun is unaspected. Not a common occurrence. The Sun is parallel Jupiter – there's your Jupiterian influence of the highs and lows. Notice what we said earlier – the Jupiter is thrown in for the mania and the Saturn for the lows. So you want to see both for manic depression. And another aspect you might not notice. You know Neptune has a lot to do with alcoholism. Neptune is contra-parallel the Ascendant. So now we're getting the Neptune influence, which you wouldn't see unless you look at declinations.

There's a cardinal T-square of Mars Uranus Pluto. This is not exactly a happy T-square. And it's angular making it more powerful. So there's a lot of aggression to over-come and a lot of problems. You could almost look at this chart as schizophrenic. And there are a lot of midpoint combinations:

Saturn = Sun/Neptune
inhibitions through illness or physical disability, emotional afflictions, illness through mental and emotional suffering.

Neptune = Sun/Ascendant
the inclination to get angry or upset easily.

Sun = Saturn/MC
lack of courage to face life, insufficient powers of defense in regard to other people, emotional depression, etc.

So this was a manic depressive alcoholic and now let's just look at the other chart of a manic depressive and see if we see some similar indications. This is the Manic

Depressive (Female) with 3 Taurus rising. Neptune is conjunct the Descendant and opposite the Ascendant – moodiness, dreaminess, disappointment, disillusionment. Mercury conjunct Pluto – nervous irritation. Jupiter conjunct Neptune – there's the elation, that up and down feeling.

Venus = Saturn/Pluto
a love of solitude, delusion, estrangement, alienation, asceticism.

Mars = Moon/Pluto
great changes of mood, easy excitability.

Jupiter = Saturn/Pluto
difficulty caused through illness.

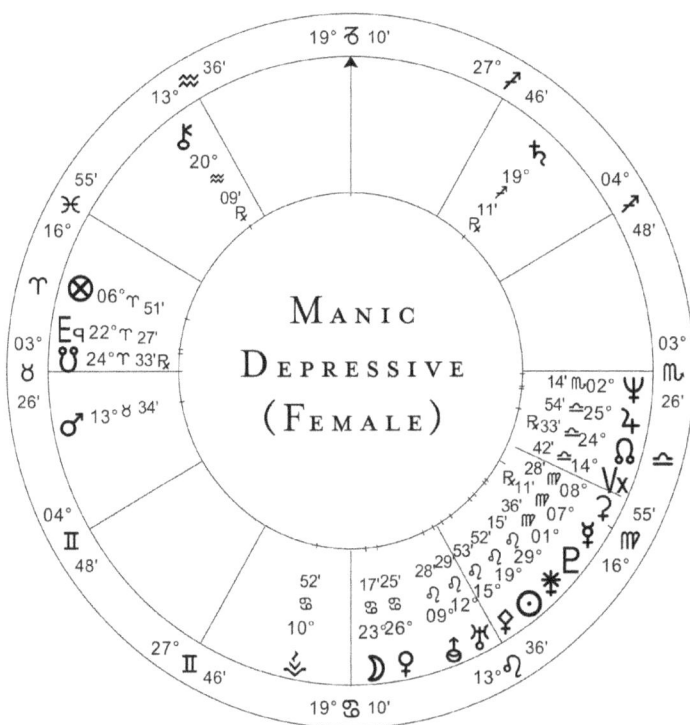

MANIC DEPRESSIVE (FEMALE)

Audience: For the manic depressive (Female), the only planet that is elevated is Saturn.

DC: Yes, Saturn is elevated and everything else is below the horizon. Very internalized.
Uranus = Mercury/MC
emotional and mental irritability, getting easily excited. Then there's some more. Getting restless and excited
Ascendant = Moon/Uranus.
Neptune = Moon/Uranus
lack of energy, weakness.

The midpoints really add to the picture. You can see highs and lows without doing the midpoints. You've got Moon square Jupiter. That's highs and lows – exaggerating everything out of proportion. And the Mercury Pluto conjunction can go from one extreme to the other. And Jupiter Neptune can be poor judgment. Then I noticed there were four close conjunctions in the chart. Four different sets of conjunctions – I think that splits your personality a little. When you're looking at a chart for mental instability, you're searching for something that points to a lack of integration which you see here.

Now look at the manic depressive chart with 16 Aries rising (Manic Depressive Female). Here's another example where the two elevated planets are Saturn and Jupiter – manic depression. So there you have that on and off again type. The Moon is parallel to Uranus which you wouldn't notice unless you look at the declinations. So there's a Moon Uranus component, which is over-excitability. Then you have Moon square Neptune, which we know can be chaotic or unstable. Obviously, these planets can also indicate psychic ability, but when you're looking at a chart to find mental health significators, you tend to talk more about these planets in terms of mental instability. And we are focusing more on the negative parts of the chart.

Moon in Leo square Neptune I thought was interesting. That could be highs and lows. Sun conjunct Mercury in the 12th house in Pisces. That definitely could be depression. And also Saturn is in Capricorn. We've got both positive and negative aspects.

MIDPOINTS:

Moon = Saturn/Uranus
strong emotional tensions and strain, states of depression and despondency.

Moon = Venus/Saturn
emotional inhibitions, emotional depression from unsatisfied love.

Venus = Saturn/Nodes
the inability to express one's feelings or emotions, a lack of adaptability.

Mars = Moon/Uranus
lack of self-control.

Uranus = Sun/Saturn
fluctuating attitude toward life, emotional tension.

Saturn = Moon/Jupiter
the inability to be happy.

Saturn = Mercury/Neptune
dark thoughts, pessimistic outlook, inhibitions in thinking.

And there were more. Here was a case where the mental instability wasn't as obvious until I started compiling all the midpoints from Ebertin that were mostly difficult combinations. I do midpoints on some of the charts that I interpret, and I might only come up with one of these midpoints. We all go through bad days. When you get ten of them that describe emotional instability, you know there's something wrong.

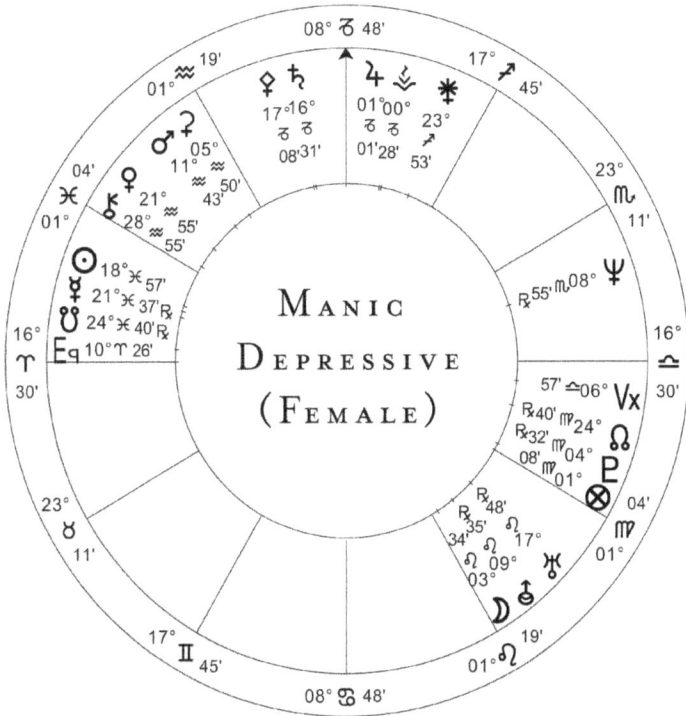

MANIC

DEPRESSIVE

(FEMALE)

Audience: What orb do you use?

DC: I'll go up to two degrees and maybe that's wide, but it works. I set the computer at 1½ degrees and 2 degrees for the personal points.

Now we can look at Howard Hughes who is a prime example of paranoia. And what aspects did I say described paranoia? Mercury Pluto. If you look at Howard Hughes' chart, we have a Mercury Pluto opposition. He had great wealth. You know what the two planets of great wealth are? Jupiter and Pluto and they're elevated. Do you see that?

HOWARD HUGHES

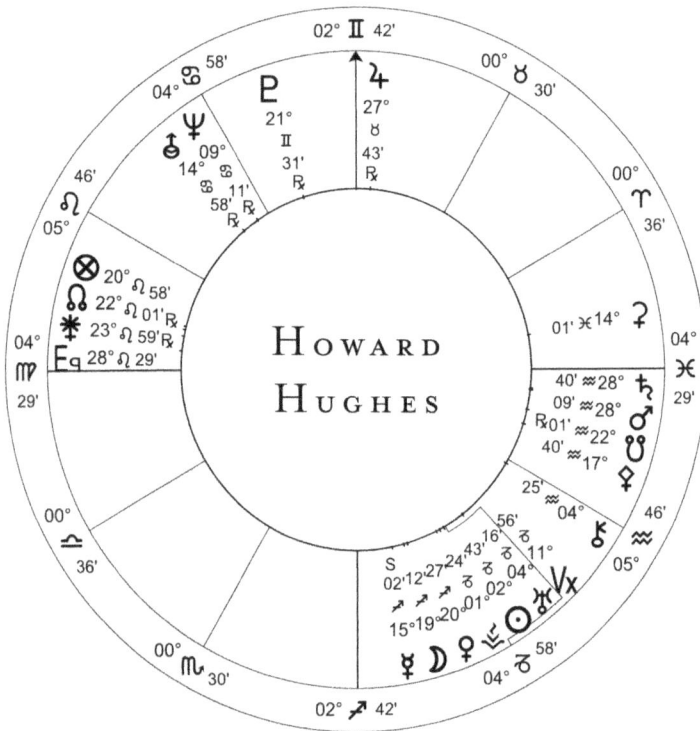

I thought that was interesting as he was immensely wealthy. Now he was paranoid about germs and everything else. What's the rising sign? Virgo. If you're going to be worried about germs, you're going to find some Virgo. And then he was compulsive and obsessive. What planets have to do with being compulsive and obsessive? Among others I think Mars Saturn. There's a Mars Saturn conjunction. Virgo can be a bit compulsive too.

Audience: He'll do it his way also.

DC: Right. And what you just said would also be the fact that he has a Sun Uranus conjunction. So we're adding on more. There's always something unusual or odd with Sun Uranus. I think many astrologers have Sun Uranus aspects too. I have Sun Uranus semisquare in my chart. I don't think we'd be studying astrology if we didn't have something with Uranus in our charts, but it could also be Neptune. So it's not that unusual to have it. In his case we're adding things up. And he's got Saturn opposite the Ascendant, which could cause withdrawal among other things. Mercury is retrograde. So he would internalize a lot. Mars conjunct Saturn can be compulsiveness and obsessiveness, inconstancy and extremes and also 00 degrees Scorpio is on the third house cusp. This puts a sign of extremes on a mental house. Mercury Pluto I thought could be paranoia. Virgo is rising. And the ruler of the chart, which is another important point, is Mercury, which is opposite Pluto. So the Mercury Pluto opposition is stronger because it involves the ruler of the chart. And they are both angular.

Here are some of his midpoints.

Moon = Jupiter/Neptune
little sense of reality, instability.

Moon = Uranus/MC
a frequent change of mood, the tendency to get upset easily.

Moon = Neptune/MC
the tendency to revel in fanciful imaginings, a misinterpretation of observations and perceptions.

And he was pretty far gone at the end. He may have been taking too many drugs.

Uranus = Sun/Neptune
a suddenly emerging weakness or illness. He didn't start out like this. An inner emotional crisis.

I didn't do anything predictive. That could be a whole other topic – looking at when these people got sick or had psychotic episodes.

MC = Saturn/Ascendant
the inclination to feel depressed, oppressed, inhibited, frustrated or slighted by others. Suffering from other people's actions.

Also there is Jupiter square Saturn – inconstancy. And Mars square Jupiter – exaggerating things out of proportion.

I looked up "paranoia" in *The Rulership Book* by Rex Bills[2]. Neptune he said or in parentheses Saturn is paranoia. So in this case I think it's Saturn.

Audience: I think it has something to do with his fourth house. He was so paranoid about leaving his home.

DC: Right. He never left that room in Las Vegas.

Audience: Where did he get his money from?

DC: Aviation. And he was a film producer.

Audience: Oil. From the family.

Audience: I've studied both the lives of Mike Wallace and Dick Cavett and both of them have had very stable and long marriages. I think Mike Wallace was married 40 something years.

DC: Maybe that's the Capricorn part (in Dick Cavett). It gives stability.

We have one more chart and that's the multiple personality chart. I saw that Neptune rising and that's really what struck me. There weren't that many midpoints that I came up with.

Saturn = Jupiter/Ascendant
inhibitions in personal development.

Uranus = Sun/Mercury
incoherent and erratic thinking.

The Moon squares the Ascendant. At first I didn't think it was that important. It can signify mood changes, but that's true of a lot of people. Then I realized the Moon is elevated and square Neptune and both are conjunct angles. As previously mentioned, Moon Neptune in hard aspect can lead to chaotic or unstable emotions as well as the need for escape. I had also mentioned that multiple personalities may have been the victims of child abuse. The Sun is in the 8th house of sex and manipulation square Pluto which could represent a forceful situation involving a male. This chart came out of a databank. And I wondered if it could just be the Neptune rising; is it that strong? I included this chart as I wanted to have a variety of charts. Does anyone have any comments on this chart?

Audience: I see lots of squares including Mars. You have the Moon Neptune and the Mars square Jupiter.

DC: Moon Neptune will definitely cause problems with the self and a lack of clarity. I've seen so-called normal people with Moon Neptune aspects, and they are very psychic and also can be emotionally confused or even unstable at times. The Mars square Jupiter could exaggerate the Moon Neptune aspect. And the Moon is also square the Ascendant which can make a person changeable.

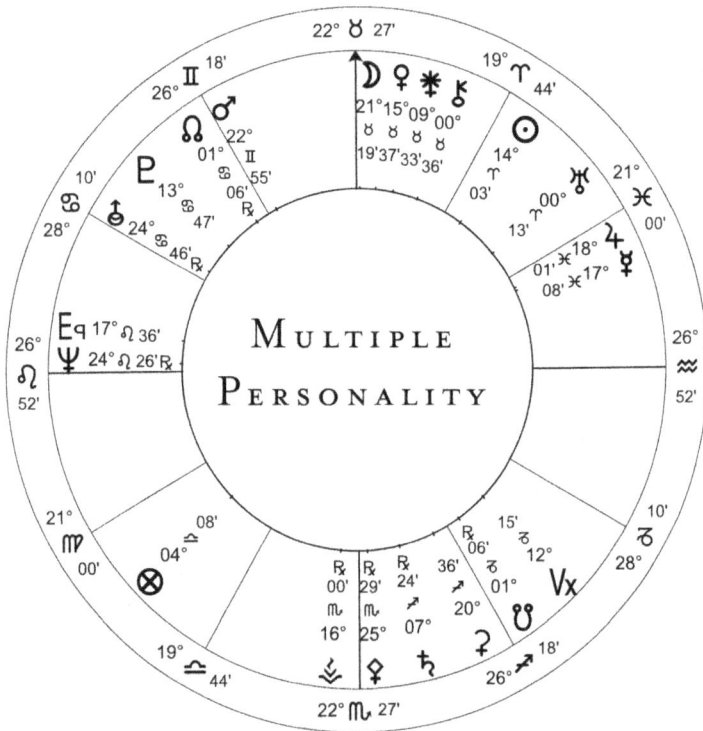

MULTIPLE PERSONALITY

I just didn't think the significators stood out like the other charts we did. I thought the schizophrenics stood out especially when you saw the Sun Uranus Neptune in both the charts; then you know it's a difficult combination.

Audience: I have a question about a lot of sextiles. There's a Mars to Neptune and the Moon Venus. So that gives them opportunities.

DC: The sextiles ease some of the problems and offer opportunities in life. I also think there may be something with the Sun, Moon and the Ascendant. Because you always want to look to see how the Sun, Moon and Ascendant combine so you can see how integrated you are. Sun in Aries, Moon in Taurus, and Leo rising. So the Taurus Moon doesn't fit in well with all that fire. It's like going in a different direction. You need one thing but you act another way. That's a difficult combination – an Aries Sun and a Taurus Moon. Because there's a fight within yourself right there. Adjacent signs don't always have a lot in common. The Aries doesn't want to stop and needs adventure, but that Moon in Taurus has got to have that security.

We went through all nine charts. And I have given you a lot of significators. There are more topics you could do in a lecture like this such as suicide or drug addiction as well as other mental disorders. Chapter Six has some information on addiction.

Audience: The Chiron Moon could indicate a problem.

DC: I'm still learning about Chiron. I'm watching it more in transit. When JFK Jr's plane went down he had Chiron square Chiron by transit and remember he was wounded (his leg). He also had Pluto transit square Pluto almost to the minute. And there were other indications in the progressions. I found that fascinating. Pluto was opposing his tenth house and natally he had Pluto square the MC. He was wounded. He shouldn't have been flying with that bad foot. That would be the Chiron influence.

Audience: What kind of advice could you give to families with these types of charts?

DC: Well, what can you say to be optimistic? I think the individuals need to have therapy. An astrologer cannot solve these problems. When I see people with various health problems in the chart I advise them to see specific health practitioners. For example, I will tell someone to go see a nutritionist if need be. I know a lot about nutrition, but I am not a nutritionist. If someone is suffering with depression, they need psycho-therapy or therapy. We may be able to point out problems to a client. For example, telling a client that their chart shows a tendency to depression. If you're not a trained therapist anymore than I'm a physician, send them to the people who can help them. As astrologers we can very quickly see problems. Unless you're trained in something, I think you're playing with fire.

This wasn't a medically oriented medical astrology lecture, but when I lecture on medical astrology one of the first things I say is don't try to diagnose. The condition could be one of many things shown in a chart. Remember in Chapter Two the three cases with a Jupiter Saturn conjunction. All three had different types of health issues. So, just be an astrologer, but don't try to be something else unless you're trained for it. People take you very seriously, and you don't want to get in over your head.

Audience: I've heard people talk about depression but they can focus.

DC: I think Saturn or Capricorn allows you to function. You can function despite being depressed.

Audience: I know depressives who can't work.

DC.: Maybe they have a work problem. I also think you have to look for ambition in a chart. Desire.

Audience: Medication is one answer.

DC: Yes, that helps some people. First you have to realize you have a problem and go for help. A lot of people function being depressed. They don't know what a happy day is. They function; they work. But inside they're very unhappy. They may need spiritual guidance. But we can't do that for them. I don't think so anyway.

REFERENCES

1. Berkow, Robert, M.D., Beers, Mark, M.D., Fletcher, Andrew, M.D.: *The Merck Manual of Medical Information Home Edition,* Merck Research Laboratories, Whitehouse Station, NJ, 1997.

2. Bills, Rex E.: *The Rulership Book,* Macoy Publishing & Masonic Supply Co., Inc., Richmond, Virginia, 1976.

3. Carter, C.E.O.: *An Encyclopaedia Of Psychological Astrology,* The Theosophical Publishing House Ltd., London, England, 1963.

4. Cornell, H.L.: *Encyclopaedia Of Medical Astrology,* Samuel Weiser, Inc., York Beach, Maine, 1972.

5. Davidson, William: *Davidson's Medical Astrology,* Astrological Bureau, Monroe, New York, 1979.

6. Ebertin, Reinhold: *Astrological Healing The History And Practice Of Astromedicine,* Samuel Weiser, Inc., York Beach, Maine, 1989.

7. Ebertin, Reinhold: *The Combination Of Stellar Influences,* Ebertin-Verlag, Aalen, Germany, 1972.

8. Harvey, Ronald: *Mind & Body In Astrology,* L.N. Fowler & Co., Ltd., Essex, England, 1983. (Information cited from p.21.)

9. Mann, A.T.: *Astrology And The Art Of Healing,* Unwin Paperbacks, London, England, 1989.

10. Ridder-Patrick, Jane: *A Handbook Of Medical Astrology,* Arkana, London, England, 1990.

11. Sakoian, Frances & Acker, Louis S., *The Astrologer's Handbook,* Harper & Row, New York. 1973. (Information cited from p. 191.)

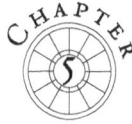

CHAPTER 5

Rebalancing with the Elements and Modes

This chapter teaches you how to find and analyze the elements and the modes in the natal chart. It also includes some information on the signs in relation to medical astrology. Cures for an imbalance of an element or a mode are given. Example charts are used to see the modes and elements in action.

I'm going to discuss using the elements and the modes to balance your health. Ever since I started studying medical astrology I was always interested in the effects of the elements and the modes. And I once read that the body is so finely tuned that even the slightest imbalance can lead to a health problem. We don't realize how finely tuned out bodies are. And it can be the slightest thing going wrong which can lead to ill health. You can use the elements and the modes to describe personality characteristics, but I'm going to explain their use both in terms of personality and in terms of health.

There are two useful books that could give you some information on the elements and the modes in terms of health. *A Guide to Natural Health* (Llewellyn) by Jonathan Keyes is full of information on the modes or quadruplicities: cardinal, fixed and mutable and the elements fire, earth, air and water in terms of health. Then my last book *Managing Your Health and Wellness* (Llewellyn) has a section on the elements and modes. And in Appendix A of that book is a lot of nutritional information on what might benefit you if you have a particular health problem. I gathered my information from many sources that are listed in the Bibliography of that book.

So let's begin with an explanation of how to determine your elements and modes in terms of points. I'm also going to give you the points for the charts used, but I will first use one chart as an example. So how do you use points when using the elements and the modes? First of all, I thought it was interesting because Jonathan Keyes uses the same point system that I use except he doesn't include the Nodes. So I saw that I wasn't the only one using this particular point system.

Do you know what a point system is? You've got to give the Sun a certain amount of points, the Moon a certain amount of points and so on. Well, you can go one for one (one point for each planet plus the Ascendant and MC) which I also do, but if you really want to emphasize the personal points in the chart you can give the Sun, the Moon and the Ascendant 4 points each. You can give Mercury, Venus and Mars 3 points each. Jupiter, Saturn and the North Node get 2 points each. Uranus, Neptune and Pluto get 1 point each, because so many people have planets in their sign placement since they move so slowly. And the ruler of the Ascendant receives 2 points.

This system was taught to me when I was first learning astrology. And I'm going to use this system when I talk to you about all the example charts. You don't have to use this system. You might like to use a system that gives two points for the Sun, Moon and Ascendant and 1 point for everything else. Whatever system you want to use that will show you what's going on in a chart is fine. You are looking for too much or an emphasis in an element or a mode or a lack or deficiency in an element or mode. Too much of an element can sometimes lead to a health problem; not enough of an element sometimes can lead to a health problem caused by an imbalance in the body. There are also personality traits based on asking: Are you very cardinal? Are you very fixed? Are you very mutable? And those also affect your health.

Let's illustrate the point system using Kurt Cobain's chart. This is a good example and as you probably know he committed suicide. And his chart is imbalanced in terms of the modes and elements. His Sun is in Pisces which is a mutable sign. Pisces is a water sign. The Sun gets 4 points. So you have 4 points for water and 4 points for mutability. The Moon is in Cancer which is a cardinal water sign. 4 for cardinal, 4 for water. The Ascendant is in Virgo which is a mutable earth sign, 4 for earth and 4 for mutable. Now we are going to use three points for Mercury, Venus and Mars. Mercury is in Pisces so we have 3 points for water and 3 points for mutability. Venus is in Pisces. 3 points for water; 3 points for mutability. Mars is in Scorpio – a fixed water sign. So we have 3 points for water and 3 points for fixed. Now we are going to do 2 points each for Jupiter, Saturn and the North Node. Now remember you don't have to use this system, but this is the system I am using now. Jonathan Keyes doesn't use the Nodes in this point system. So you can take it or leave it with the Nodes, but I do find them useful in medical astrology. Hard aspects to the Nodes can indicate a health disorder based on the sign such as Saturn square the Nodes in Gemini could point to a respiratory disorder.

Jupiter is in Cancer so now we have 2 points for cardinal, 2 points for water. Saturn is in Pisces. 2 for mutability, 2 for water. And the North Node is in Taurus. 2 for earth, 2 for fixed. If you are a beginner you have to think through this. If you are not a beginner, it's not a difficult process. Uranus, Neptune and Pluto get 1 point each. Uranus is in Virgo and Virgo is mutable earth. 1 for earth, 1 for mutable. Neptune is in Scorpio which is fixed water. 1 for fixed, 1 for water. And Pluto is in Virgo which is 1 for mutable and 1 for earth. The ruler of the Ascendant is Mercury in Pisces which gets 2 points. 2 for mutable and 2 for water. Now you add them up. See the following table. Mutability which I will discuss can have a mental component. It has other characteristics, but it has a mental factor to it and you see the large number of points in mutability. You see a complete imbalance here. And what else do you see or not see? You don't see any fire or any air.

Kurt Cobain					
Fire		0	Cardinal	4, 2	6
Earth	4, 2, 1, 1	8	Fixed	3, 2, 1	6
Air		0	Mutable	4, 4, 3, 3, 2, 1, 1, 2	20
Water	4, 4, 3, 3, 3, 2, 2, 1, 2	24			

With this system you can see if someone is missing an element or has too much of an element. I'll discuss what you can do about an imbalance with the elements. Now supposedly if you have a strong Mars in your chart, it makes up for a lack of fire. If you have a strong Saturn in your chart, it makes up for a lack of earth. If you have a strong Uranus in your chart, it's supposed to make up for a lack of air. And if you have a strong Neptune in your chart,

KURT COBAIN

it is supposed to make up for a lack of water in the chart. All the years I've been using this system, I still wonder. You have to weigh this information with everything else in the chart. Can an emphasized planet made up for a lack of an element? Kurt Cobain has Uranus rising which would have helped the lack of air. And certainly a lot of mutability is very mental.

This point system is one of the ways to determine what you have in your chart in terms of the modes or quadruplicities. And you would say that Kurt Cobain was prone to mutable types of illnesses. It is important to always understand that medical astrology is based on the crosses. You don't just have a problem in Aries. It could show up in Libra, but it manifests as Aries. You have to think in terms of crosses: cardinal, fixed and mutable. I'm going to discuss cardinal, fixed and mutable also in terms of personality. Then from the personality characteristics you ask what is the illness as a result of having an abundance of an element or mode or not enough of an element or mode, and what are the cures for it?

Audience: What planet did you say makes up for a lack of air?

DC: Uranus.

Again, this rule of a planet making up for a lack of an element sometimes works and other times doesn't. I always look for an elevated planet or a planet that stands out in the chart to make up for a lack of something.

Audience: Is the planet strong based on what house it's in or what sign it is in?

DC: It's strong if it's elevated, angular or the ruler of the chart. You could use those rules.

Audience: Couldn't this intense mutability in this chart make up to some extent for a lack of air?

DC: The excess mutability caused him to become mentally distraught or mentally off in some way. He did commit suicide. So, no, I don't look at it that way. Also, the air element has to do with oxygen and circulation in the body. I don't think an excess of a mode makes up for a lack of an element in terms of medical astrology. It could be true in natal astrology interpretation.

Audience: What about the houses such as air houses, etc?

DC: Yes and no. That's the problem. I haven't found that when something is so lacking that a house emphasis totally makes up for it, but at the same time it can help. Like everything else in astrology; you have to experiment and see what works or what doesn't work for you. Which takes me to the next rule. There are cardinal, fixed and mutable types of illnesses and when you start to learn medical astrology, you learn that Aries rules the head, Taurus rules the neck and you just continue with the signs throughout your body. That part is fairly simple. You get to the feet and you have Pisces. When I was first learning medical astrology, one of the ways I determined proneness to a certain type of disease or mode was the point system that I just illustrated with Kurt Cobain's chart.

The other method is to look for malefics afflicting the angles which I've touched on earlier in the book. I learned this method from *Essentials of Medical Astrology* by Dr. Harry Darling. Let's say Saturn is in a hard aspect to your MC and your MC is in Sagittarius, then you would say that you have a proneness to mutable types of diseases. This is because Sagittarius is a mutable sign. Take your Ascendant, IC, Descendant and MC – houses 1, 4, 7 or 10. Is there an outer planet – Saturn, Uranus, Neptune, Pluto or Mars making a difficult aspect to the cusp of house 1, 4, 7 or 10. If the answer is yes, what sign is it? For example, my MC is in Sagittarius. That means that you can have a problem involving the meaning of that particular cross – which in this case is the mutable cross since

Sagittarius is a mutable sign. I find there are two ways to see what crosses are activated in the chart. One way is to do the point system; the other way is to use the angles of the chart. Dr. Harry Darling considered malefics to the angles to indicate what he called first-degree proneness to illness in the quadrature indicated.

Let's take another example. You are Taurus rising and Saturn is conjunct your Ascendant. You have 1st degree proneness to illness in the fixed cross because Taurus is fixed, and it is being afflicted by a malefic. Consider cardinal, fixed and mutable types of illnesses. Think that way first and then break the information down into more specifics. So think crosses.

Audience: Hard aspects?

DC: Hard aspects of the outer planets but also Mars which is not an outer planet. Hard aspects of the outer planets plus Mars are used. For advanced astrologers use the Vertex which is considered the third angle of the chart. Afflictions to the Vertex work also in determining an afflicted cross. You look at your chart and say, "I've got Neptune afflicting my IC. My IC is in Scorpio. I am prone to fixed-cross types of illnesses." If you don't have malefics to the angles, but you have malefics to other parts of the chart, it's not as serious. The seriousness is the angularity. Angularity makes it more severe.

Audience: If you have Mars conjunct the Vertex?

DC: What's your Vertex in?

Audience: It's in Libra.

DC: Then you could have problems related to the cardinal cross.

This method of looking at malefics to the angles works. Until I began using it, I had a lot of trouble understanding medical astrology and in understanding what was serious and what wasn't in the chart or in understanding why such and such happened to someone. I didn't think you could tell. And then when I learned this method, I went "Aha. It works." This is what you're prone to. Combine it with the points and the other methods I've described in this book, and you've got a way of seeing your weaknesses.

Audience: What's more important in determining the cause? The amount of mutability?

DC: No, I would say malefics to the angles.

It's not always that simple. Sometimes you can see all the crosses active. But you have to determine at what point in life disease may manifest. I think the answer is to be aware. We all know people with serious health problems. You're going to see that malefics hitting the angles are the serious issues in life. So if you have problems involving cadent houses, they will not be as serious. It could be something that will come and go. Some people have more difficult charts than other people. And the problems seem to be shown by malefics to angles – the seriousness of the problem. Of course, difficult planetary combinations such as a Grand Cross can also indicate difficulty.

So when I'm looking at a chart I'm using points, but I'm also looking at malefics to the angles. And when you look at a chart you say to yourself, "Oh, this person has an emphasis in mutability and water. What's the mutable water sign? Pisces." Sometimes an emphasis won't be the same as the person's Sun sign. When you're doing a regular read-ing and trying to determine a person's personality traits, you might be doing the chart of someone in a particular sign. And they turn out to have an emphasis such as Pisces even though that is not their Sun sign. So I will mention to the person that yes, you were born a Scorpio, but you've got a big emphasis in such and such. You take the highest points in the modes and the highest points in the elements and put them together and you've got a personality trait for the person. It won't always be their Sun sign. It was in the case of Kurt Cobain with his mutable water emphasis which equals Pisces and he did have his Sun in Pisces.

Audience: Where do you get those numbers – the 20 and the 24.

DC: I added up the planets in water and got 24, and I added up the mutable planets and got 20.

Audience: I have a question on the crosses. When you're looking at aspects to the MC for example, does the aspect have to be a square or can it be another angle?

DC: The aspect should be a square, opposition or conjunc-tion. Harry Darling did not use the semisquare or the sesquiquadrate in determining afflictions to the angles. He only used the square, opposition and the conjunction.

Audience: But the quincunx is a classic aspect.

DC: I know. Here is another thing. If it works for you, then use it. Astrologers rarely go by rigid rules. I don't use the quincunx when I'm looking for afflictions to the angles.

I do use the quincunx when I'm doing a chart reading. But when I'm asking myself if this person has a problem with a particular cross, I just use the conjunction, square or opposition. The quincunx is one of those on again, off again aspects so that may be why it is not used in this method of determining afflictions to the angles. And by the way you are looking at all four angles – the Ascendant, Descendant, MC, and IC. And also the Vertex.

Audience: Do you use the conjunction?

DC: A conjunction if it's Mars, Saturn, Uranus, Neptune or Pluto.

Audience: So you are just using the Ptolemaic aspects. Also the trines and the sextiles to see if there is anything helpful.

DC: Oh, sure. I use the sextiles and the trines to show what's helpful in the chart. I also use the semi-square and sesquiquadrate as part of the reading as a whole. When I'm giving a reading, I'm looking for strengths and weaknesses in a chart. So you want to try to show people the positive parts of their charts, but at the same time you don't want to minimize the problems either. The biggest problem with medical astrology is that you can upset people. You upset yourself. You think you're going to get every disease you study just like when you were a beginner in astrology, you knew you were going to have a disaster next week because you were getting a difficult transit. You take it so seriously and then years go by. Wait a minute. It's not quite like that. Well, it's the same with medical astrology. You can see the most difficult combinations in a chart. It doesn't manifest because you have to take into account lifestyle and hereditary. At the same time, you don't want to ignore that your chart shows a tendency to heart disease, for example. Maybe you should be on a heart-healthy diet. You have to really know how to talk to people.

Audience: Is it too soon to ask a question about timing?

DC: Well, I think timing is interpreting your transits and progressions, etc. In fact I don't even use the word timing. I use the word "stress" and also the word "vitality." You will have a period of either lowered vitality or stress coming up. You just can't lay trips on people. And when people are very ill, you do anything you can, even if it's a few years away, and find a good progression or transit so you can give them a time of improvement. I did this for someone who had Epstein Barr Virus Syndrome. I have an article I wrote on Epstein Barr Virus Syndrome in an old NCGR Journal that was dedicated to medical astrology. The subject was a doctor and I saw 10 years down the road an improvement. And it did take 10 years for him to improve or to be free of the disease. That is a very serious disease. He had to give up his medical practice. So whatever you can see that can give people hope – you can look at the progressed Moon for periods of improvement. You'll feel better such and such a month; you may have less vitality in such and such a month. Whatever you can do. You should help people. Don't let them leave a reading thinking it's hopeless. It's over. In medical readings you can be dealing with people with very serious diseases. Let's get back to the subject at hand.

Audience: Some days I feel good; some days I feel bad.

DC: Well, that can be the daily transits of the Moon, biorhythms, transits to your Sun. Let's start with Cardinality.

CARDINAL MODE

An example of a chart with excess cardinality is Nancy Hastings. Her chart can be found in Chapter Two where it was first discussed. Let me give you her numbers. As mentioned previously, Nancy Hastings wrote two books on progressions. She was a well-known astrologer and she died several years ago of cancer. It was pretty tragic. She has the following points:

Fire: 5
Earth: 12
Air: 6
Water: 9
Cardinal: 23
Fixed: 1
Mutable: 8

So she is an example of a chart with a cardinal emphasis. Cardinal types of people are very willful, very wired, sometimes very hyper. Cardinal people can have Type A behavior. Some health practitioners feel Type A is prone to coronary heart disease. Others disagree with this theory.

THE FOLLOWING IS FROM WIKIPEDIA:

"**Type A** individuals can be described as impatient, excessively time-conscious, insecure about their status, highly competitive, over-ambitious, business-like, hostile, aggressive, incapable of relaxation in taking the smallest issues too seriously; and are somewhat disliked for the way that they're always rushing and demanding other people to serve to their standards of satisfaction. They are often high and over-achieving workaholics who multi-task, drive themselves with deadlines, and are unhappy about the smallest of delays. Because of these characteristics, **Type A** individuals are often described as "stress junkies." **Type B** individuals, in contrast, are described as patient, relaxed, and easy-going. There is also a **Type AB** mixed profile for people who cannot be clearly categorized."

Cardinal people tend to get acute types of disease. Each type of disease is represented by the quadruplicity. So cardinal is acute, fixed is chronic and mutable can be recurring. I'll come back to that. Mutable can be acute also. Since cardinal types like action; they also want to get results immediately if they get ill. They don't want to wait. They want to know right away what's wrong and what to do about it. Now *The American Book of Nutrition and Medical Astrology* by Eileen Nauman describes the root causes of disease. She says that the root cause of cardinal types of diseases are the kidneys and the gallbladder. So if you have a problem in cardinality in your chart, then you can nourish or avoid putting a strain on the kidneys or gallbladder. Now when I say nourish, you can nourish any part of your body. I've seen this word used in books that I read that say nourish the part of your body that is weak. You take foods or supplements to nourish the kidneys or the gallbladder or you can avoid substances that are harmful to those areas. It's both. Avoidance and nourishing.

People who have cardinality emphasized need to recognize their limits. They tend to push forth too much. They tend to annoy other people because they get in their way.

They need boundaries and they need to take responsibility for their own actions as they cause a lot of their own problems. Cardinality can be very fast energy. Now the parts of the body which have to do with cardinality are the head – there's Aries; the kidneys – there's Libra; the skin and bones – that's Capricorn, the stomach – there's Cancer. Both my introductory book – *How to Give an Astrological Health Reading* – and my previous book *Managing Your Health and Wellness* have information on the signs and their relation to the parts of the body. The latest book was written more for the layperson. I've tried to simplify the study of medical astrology even more than in my first book. Both books take you through the parts of the body.

Audience: Cardinality is the head?

DC: Yes, so you've got the head, kidneys, the stomach, skin and bones. So if you know your signs you know that Aries refers to the head, Capricorn to skin, bones and nails, and Libra rules the kidneys. This is simplified but it can be used as a general guide. And then you've got Cancer for the stomach. Cancer also rules the chest cage. Cancer rules coverings in the body. It also rules containers which is why it rules the womb and the stomach and the breasts. You start to learn what these signs rule and where they fall in the body. And with cardinality you can experience gallbladder problems, heartburn, high blood pressure.

So for people with an emphasis in cardinality you need relaxing and soothing foods, and you need to nourish yourself as you can always be in a hurry. You need nourishing food. If you could do meditation, yoga or tai chi that would be helpful. Taking relaxing herbs such as chamomile, lemon balm, skullcap and possibly digestive herbs and spices such as garlic, fennel and basil can help. You should also eat more whole grains and vegetables, small amounts of meat and fish and if you are a vegetarian, you want to include foods such as tofu, beans and nuts in your diet. You also have to be careful of too much caffeine or drugs and also sugar as you are already wired out. Drinking a lot of soda which contains caffeine and sugar could be detrimental to your health. So you want to keep these substances low in your diet.

FIXED MODE
Carl Sagan is one example of a chart with a fixed emphasis. Let me give you the numbers for him.

Fire: 5
Earth: 8
Air: 4
Water: 15
Cardinal: 2
Fixed: 22
Mutable: 8

He certainly was rigid when it came to astrology. Now, what are fixed-type people like? They can be rigid and stubborn. That's why their bodies can get stiff, and they can contract diseases like arthritis. They stick with things that are not worth sticking to. The fixed type can get stuck in a rut and needs to learn to be more flexible. The root cause of fixed type of illnesses is the colon and secondarily the thyroid. So those parts of the body need to be nourished if you have an emphasis in fixed signs. That is the one mode that can be prone to retaining toxins. The fixed emphasis also has to do with your personality – not letting go. Toxins accumulate in your body. You need to loosen up. And a lot of disease is caused by toxicity and toxic build-up in the body. And fixed problems can affect the throat – Taurus, the reproductive organs – Scorpio, eliminative organs – Scorpio, the heart – Leo, and circulation – Aquarius. Leo and Aquarius refer to the heart and circulation. That's why when you do medical astrology you think in terms of the polarities and the crosses. When you do natal astrology you're not necessarily thinking like that, but you can use an emphasis in a particular cross to describe personality. Because we all know fixed-type people.

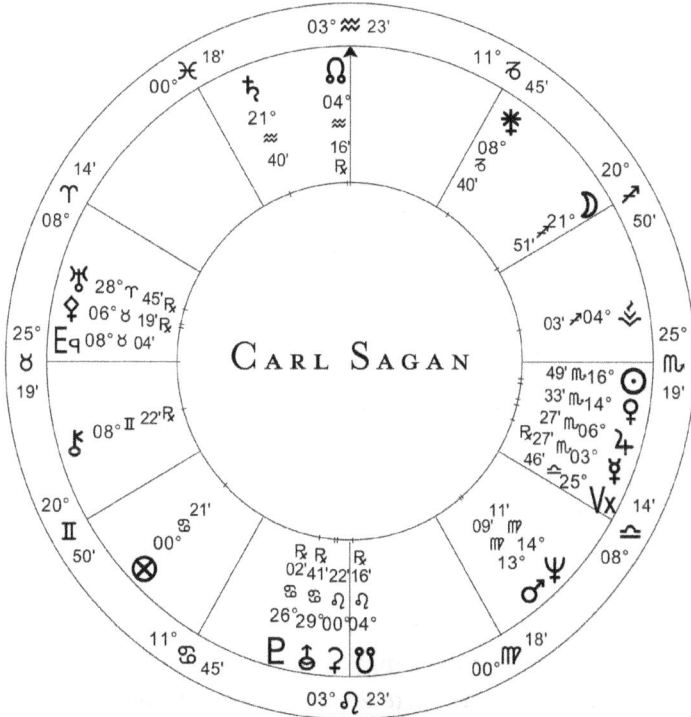

CARL SAGAN

Fixed can refer to illnesses which are cumulative. Cysts and blockages. Now, Carl Sagan had a bone marrow type of cancer that sounds more like a cardinal disease to me, but I assume the fixed means there was an accumulation of toxins in his body. (Bone marrow is ruled by the sign Cancer which is on the cardinal cross.) I think a lot of illness is cumulative. I can't always figure out why someone has a particular disease unless I spend a lot of time studying the chart. It's not always that obvious. A lot of times you can see a problem right away. That's typical of astrology.

With a fixed emphasis, you need to have variety in your diet. You could have a colon condition or a heart condition because you never change your diet. Your body changes and you have to change. There can be conditions such as blockages, cysts or tumors. All of these are fixed problems. You need to get the energy moving if you have a fixed emphasis. You should not have a lot of greasy food or heavy food. You need spices in your diet; foods that stimulates your body. So you start incorporating spices into your diet. And obviously you shouldn't try to make a lot of changes at once no matter what your problem is.

Always make changes gradually to make sure you're not ingesting something your body doesn't like. Don't run out and have a ten-spice meal until you are sure you can handle the spices. Take it gradually. A lot of fixed problems are psychological, and there can be emotional and psychological toxins that get stored in the body. Body therapies such as bioenergetics and rolfing can help. You can wear gems that also help you. There are books you can buy on gem healing but for fixed types smoky quartz and black obsidian are helpful. And occasionally going on a liquid diet or a juice diet (which should be done under supervision) can be helpful for a fixed emphasis. Eat cleansing foods such as broccoli, lettuce and lemons. Lemons are very cleansing. Herbs. Ginger and cayenne give you more heat and aid your circulation. You can have ginger tea or use more cayenne on your food.

MUTABLE MODE

An example of excess mutability is the chart of Peter Jennings. Here is the point count for his chart.

Fire: 9

Earth: 14

Air: 0 (He died of lung cancer.) And he was an announcer. Do you see how you make up for a lack of an element? And he smoked.

Water: 9

Cardinal: 7

Fixed: 10

Mutable: 15. He was in a communicative field.

Mutable personalities can be extremely versatile and adaptable. Negatively they can become very scattered and become nervous wrecks. It's what we see so much of these days – multi-tasking. You call someone and usually they are on the Internet at the same time they are talking to you. And I'm guilty of this also. And I read recently that all this multitasking is leading to illness or at least to stress. We are overtaxing our bodies. If you want to be on the Internet, then just be on the Internet. Of course if you're on the phone, it's a good time to get your dishes done. So it seems that everyone is doing six things at once. I recently read that doing something such as folding your laundry and watching television is not harmful in terms of multitasking. Talking on the phone and reading email or driving a car and talking on a cell phone at the same time is really not multitasking. It's forcing the brain to switch back and forth quickly between two activities and can be detrimental to health. It's very mutable and it's very bad for us.

Also, mutable diseases can recur. They're gone. They come back. They can also morph into something else. They start out one with one set of symptoms and end up as something else. They can linger; they can recur. The root cause of mutable types of illnesses is the lymph glands and the pancreas. Both of them. And mutable diseases are

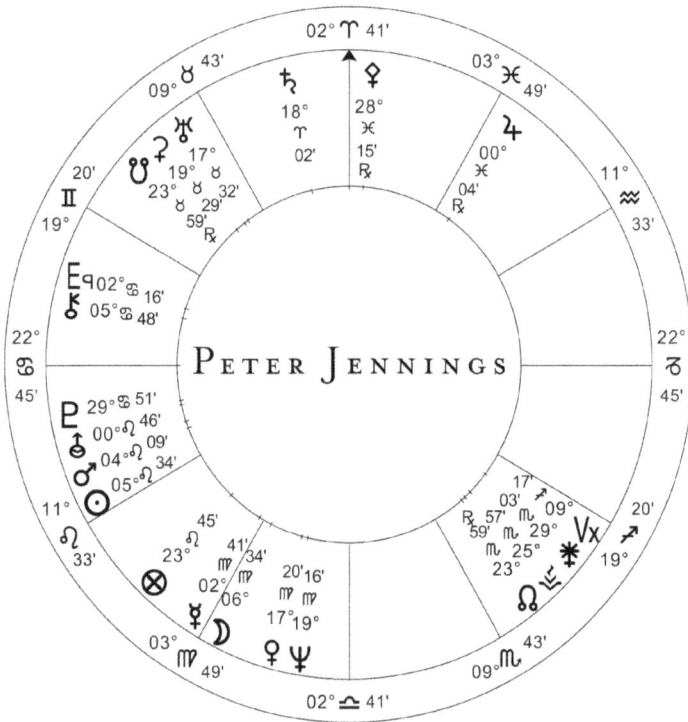

PETER JENNINGS

associated with the lungs, the intestines, nervous system and the feet. Pisces rules the feet, but it also is the ruler of the immune system. Then Gemini – lungs and nervous system; Virgo – pancreas and intestines. Sagittarius rules the hips, thighs and arteries. Virgo also has to do with the processes of discrimination and assimilation in the body.

Audience: What rules the lymph nodes?

DC: The lymph nodes are mutable and are found throughout the body and are ruled by Pisces. They are components of the lymphatic system.

Remember, I'm a medical astrologer, not a doctor. I don't always understand the body myself. I've studied books on anatomy and disease states to teach myself about the body. When I was writing my last book I realized I didn't even know exactly where the liver was in the body. I thought I'd better look it up in my anatomy book. I think a lot of medical astrology is intuitive, but you need to have some medical information. I started studying health the same time I started studying astrology which is how I ended up learning medical astrology. I certainly never claim to have anything like the knowledge of a physician, and you should go to a medical doctor for any kind of a health problem. But it's amazing what is in a chart.

Now, metabolic disorders are also associated with mutability. And disorders with a mental origin. Let me give you the numbers for Howard Hughes who is an example of someone with a mental disorder. Howard Hughes' chart was discussed in Chapter Four: Mental Aberrations in the Chart. You can find his chart there.

HOWARD HUGHES:
Fire: 18
Earth: 7
Air: 6
Water: 1
Cardinal: 6
Fixed: 9
Mutable: 17

So there's that mutable emphasis in his chart that is related to mental issues. So with mutability you never feel you have enough time; you can be scattered and nervous, and you're easily distracted. It can describe diseases of distraction, irrational fears, respiratory problems, glucose imbalance, all illnesses associated with signs on the mutable cross. So to understand this, ask yourself, what's Gemini? Respiratory. Again, you have to get some kind of beginning medical astrology book to help yourself. If you have an emphasis in mutability, you need to learn to focus your attention, finish one thing before you start something else, realize that you have the ability to recover from illnesses quickly as mutability has the ability to throw off. That's the positive part of mutability. You need grounding.

You should watch out for foods that over stimulate your nervous system. You should have grounding foods such as whole grains, tubers, some fish and meat and herbs that tone the entire system such as ginseng. Coffee, sugar, and tobacco are sometimes used as stimulants by persons with excess mutability and should be kept low because mutable types tends to run on nervous energy.

THE ELEMENTS

In *Astrology, Psychology, and the Four Elements* Stephen Arroyo discusses using the element of your Sun to build up your vitality. For example, fire signs need sunlight, earth signs need to do earthy activities such as gardening or hiking in the woods, air signs need fresh air such as found in the mountains and water signs need to be around water. If you are a water sign, going to a lake or the ocean would rejuvenate you. So could taking a bath. Everything is what you choose to do. You can't change anything if you don't take your life into your own hands.

Audience: What is air?

DC: Air is going to the mountains or having fresh circulating air around you. Earth signs should also have plants around them.

Audience: Does the element of the Moon have the same significance?

DC: The element of the Moon can have to do with health issues relevant to its sign, but it's more the Sun sign that can help rejuvenate you. You can't do everything in your chart, but I would pick the element of the Sun as it's very important.

FIRE ELEMENT

Now, the first element is fire which when it is balanced in the chart can indicate creativity and confidence. And fire thrives on excitement and you have to find a healthy way to channel the energy such as through sports or physical activity. Now, if you want to see a chart with excess fire, here are the numbers for David Crosby who had a liver transplant.

Fire: 17 and notice Mars is rising. You know he has lived a pretty hard life and did a lot of drinking.

Earth: 12

Air: 3

Water: 0

Cardinal: 9

Fixed: 14

Mutable: 9

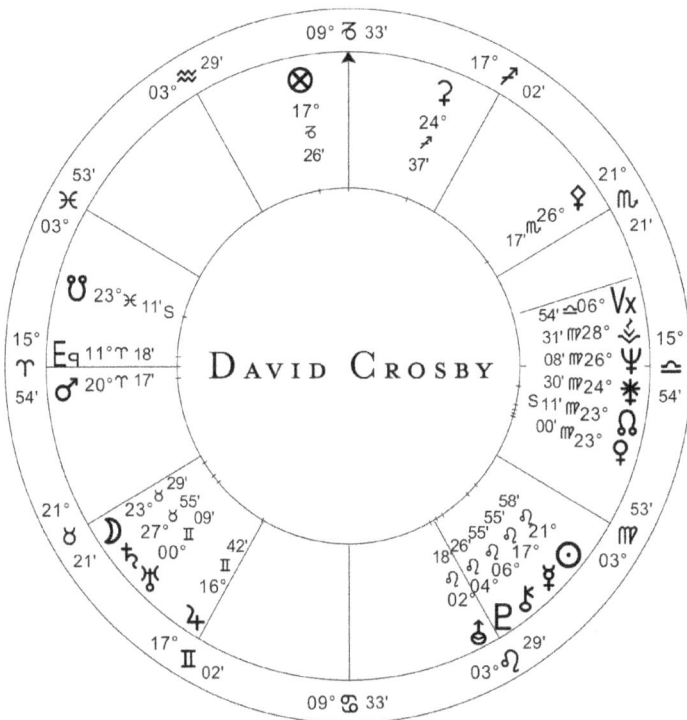

EXCESS FIRE

Those with excess fire can be angry, hot-tempered, pushy, manipulative and can burn themselves out. They seek challenges and they crave excitement. They can be hungry all the time; they can become easily dehydrated. So if you have too much fire and little water in your chart, you can have a real problem with dehydration. And you can get conditions like hepatitis, heartburn and ulcers with an excess of fire. Also gallbladder problems, skin eruptions. Even heart attacks. Digestive problems. You need to learn how to conserve your energy. You should have cold foods to tone down the fire. Bland foods tone down fire also. Sour fruits are good; raw or steamed vegetables are good. You might be able to handle sweets better than the other elements. The antidote for excess fire is water. So cold showers, cold baths, sailing, surfing, swimming. And be careful of getting too much sun and ingesting too many stimulants. You can also wear cool colors like blues and greens.

Audience: When you think of this idea that whatever your Sun sign is, it can rejuvenate you, what would rejuvenate you if your Sun is in fire?

DC: Sunlight.

Audience: What if you have too much fire?

DC: Then wear a sun screen and a big hat when you go outside. You've still got to get sunlight. It's important for your eyesight; it's gets rid of jet lag. One of the cures for jet lag is getting sunlight. And it's a source of Vitamin D. And I just think people avoid the Sun too much as they are afraid of skin cancer. Of course if you read that book *Natural Cures They Don"t Want You to Know About* by Kenneth Trudeau he says that sunscreens cause skin cancer. He says it's just another item big business want to sell you.

Audience: Let's take some contradictory information. Let's say someone has their Sun in earth but they are primarily fire.

DC: You have to think it through. And it's not something I can answer without studying the entire chart. Again, it's like everything in astrology. You have to weigh the whole chart. I spend a few hours preparing a health reading, so I would have come up with something based on my evaluation of the whole chart. In this case, their basic nature is still their Sun in earth so earth cures would not only rejuvenate them but could possibly tone down the fire.

Audience: Would it also work the other way around? For example if someone has little air in their chart, would a ceiling fan help?

DC: Yes, definitely. I haven't gotten to that yet. I was just mentioning the element of the Sun as a quick cure. Then I will give you the remedies for a lack of an element also.

So we saw David Crosby's chart is an example of excess fire and if you know his life, it does describe him. He has an incredible talent. His voice. It's interesting because he has no water. So you know how you can over compensate for a lack of an element. He became a great singer. I think when you lack an element in your chart you become that element also. It's really interesting how it works. The

Venus Neptune conjunction in his chart would also give him great sensitivity as well as artistic talent.

LOW FIRE

Madeline Kahn is an example of low fire. She died of ovarian cancer.

Fire: 1
Earth: 8
Air: 17
Water: 6
Cardinal: 12
Fixed: 1
Mutable: 19

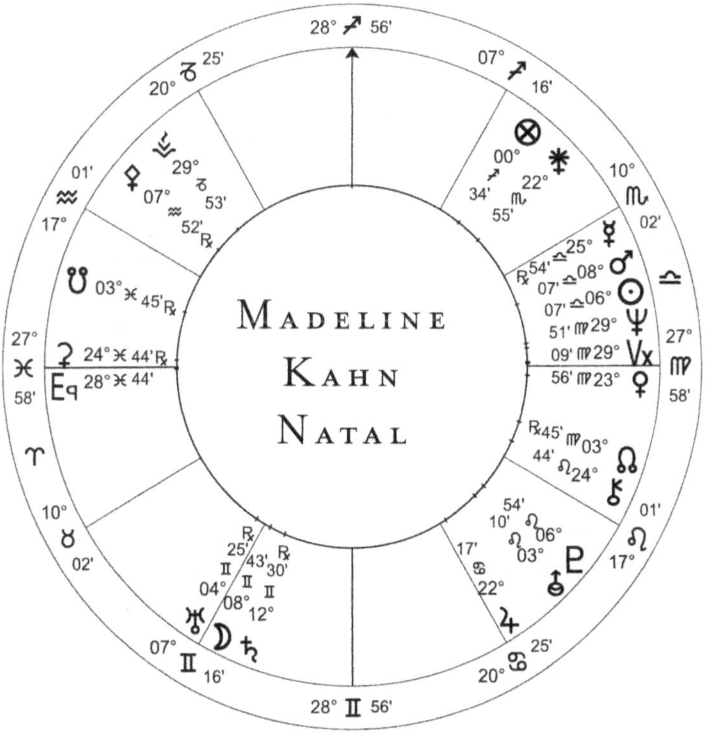

MADELINE

KAHN

NATAL

Low fire can be difficult because it can relate to poor self-esteem, low energy and poor resistance. Certainly, poor self-esteem can be an issue when you don't have a lot of fire. And when you have a lack of fire in your chart you need to do something that is not competitive, something that makes you feel good about yourself. You need an activity that makes you feel empowered. It should be an activity that gives you self-confidence. Like rollerblading. Or hiking. Biking. You don't have to do it with anybody else. When you can say to yourself, "Hey, I'm great at this." This builds up low fire in a chart as well as building up a weak Mars. With low fire, you can become depressed too easily, despondent and lack courage. Also there is the potential for poor eyesight. There can be health problems. Being overweight. Low blood pressure. And definitely poor digestion. Probably the most obvious are poor vitality and poor digestion. You can also be stiff with cold extremities with low fire.

And you don't resist or fight disease as well with low fire. So you need to apply fire. Heart and blood tonics are good. Physical exercise. Spices. Sour foods. Frequent light meals. Jane Ridder-Patrick in *A Handbook of Medical Astrology* includes a lot of information on the properties and antidotes for an imbalance of the elements. She describes fire as hot, dry and aromatic and says it can be increased by foods with these properties. Heating herbs and spices such as basil, garlic, cayenne pepper, cinnamon and ginger are useful. And aerobic exercise increases fire. And encouragement from others. One simple remedy is to light candles. That brings in fire. Or use a fireplace. Wear red or orange. Utilize gems that are red such as ruby's and garnets. If you live on the top of a mountain, play brass instruments so you won't be bothering your neighbors.

Apparently, brass instruments or listening to rousing music makes up for a lack of fire as does singing and painting. Also, develop your muscles.

EARTH ELEMENT

If earth is balanced in your chart, you're patient, you're steady, and you're grounded. And most earth signs like predictability. They don't like dealing with a lot of change. And they like job security.

Now Peter Jennings who was discussed under Mutability has an excess of the earth element. Dick Cavett also has excess of earth. He suffered with depression. His chart was discussed in Chapter 4: "Mental Aberrations in the Chart." Refer to his chart in Chapter 4. Here are his numbers:

Fire: 4
Earth: 13
Air: 3
Water: 12
Cardinal: 15
Fixed: 8
Mutable: 9

EXCESS EARTH

Too much earth can be sluggish, lethargic, depressed and slow. You may not want to accept new ideas. There can be a lack of creativity. Frozen feelings. Obsessiveness. Sometimes you can be too obsessed with your health. Also, too sedentary. You can have a stocky body and experience dryness. Too much earth is prone to heavy metal poisoning. Be aware of that. You can definitely be toxic. I think vitamin C is helpful for heavy metals. Excess earth also means you can get blockages, congestion in the body. You have a proneness to chronic conditions. You need lighter foods to counteract the heaviness of earth. Where a lack of earth type should eat potatoes and root vegetables because they are heavy foods and can also tolerate meat, it's the opposite if you have an excess of earth. You should increase spices to help stimulate your body. Consume foods that grow high such as vegetables used in salads, also sprouts. Seaweed is considered beneficial for excess earth. Dairy foods should be kept low. And fire helps to stimulate excess earth. Sports that promote agility such as ping pong and badminton counteract excess earth. Be careful of too much dry food or rich food. Yellow and orange energizes excess earth. Remember you can wear gems with the colors you need or if you're someone who has a lack of fire but doesn't like wearing red, you can buy red underwear. You can use colors in your décor such as red or orange pillows for a lack of fire and yellow and orange pillows for excess earth.

WEAK EARTH

Those with a lack of earth can be a bit spacey. They need grounding. They can be a bit out there. They don't feel like they belong. Weak earth can lose track of time and not be good at dealing with money or bank accounts. They can also be underweight. They may not be practical. Remember, these are pure meanings. No one will have all these characteristics. Health problems can be weak bones and teeth, poor skin tone. You need to get outside. You can be helped by sunshine and using oils on your body to make your skin glow such as comfrey, lavender or calendula oils. Get your feet into the mud. Go out into nature. You may have poor physical strength and poor nutrition with a lack of earth. So you need grounding techniques, heavy foods such as potatoes, squash, beets, turnips and whole grains. Just think of lighter foods if you have too much earth, heavy foods if you have a lack of earth. And walking barefoot on the earth aids weak earth types. You need very nutritious foods also. You can put cheese or butter on your vegetables if you lack earth. Massage is also beneficial. So is taking a business training course and learning money management.

AIR ELEMENT

What attributes does a person have where air is balanced in the chart? They are sociable. They have a good sense of humor. They're playful. They are light and quick and have good minds. What do we know about air signs? They like mental and intellectual stimulation. They like to be with other people. They like to socialize. They can be a bit abstract at times. And they sometimes don't handle intimacy well.

EXCESS AIR

Madeline Kahn who was discussed as an example of low fire is also an example of high air. Scott Hamilton has a decent amount of air and I wanted to give you his numbers too. See his chart and a discussion on his chart in Chapter Two: "Practical Approaches to Medical Astrology." He has to have a reasonable amount of air as he's an ice skater and has to have agility. He had testicular cancer that he overcame and had a lot of health problems as a child that stunted his growth.

Fire: 11
Earth: 8
Air: 12
Water: 1
Cardinal: 8
Fixed: 17
Mutable: 7

A person with high air can have an overactive mind and experience nervous exhaustion. Personality-wise, they can be scattered, restless, cold and anxious. Also detached. You know you're not going to get too involved in feelings even in close relationships when you have a lot of air in your chart. You don't understand your feelings until you talk about them. And you don't always listen to your body. That's another issue also with a lack of earth. You don't listen to your body. Our bodies send us messages when we eat something that doesn't agree with us, when something hurts, etc. If you listen to your body, you may be able to nip a problem in the bud. Those with a lack of earth and high air may ignore signals from their bodies. Now with high air, you can get conditions such as asthma, dry skin, brittle hair and nails, stiff joints. arthritis and thin and balding hair. Also flatulence and shooting pains in the body. You need rest and relaxation, whole grains in the diet. Deep blue and violet relax the nerves. Mineral baths are good for you. They would also be good for low earth. And root vegetables. Calming music. Air dries up water. So if you have too much air and low water, you can become thirsty and dehydrated. So water therapies and moist therapies are good. Herbal teas such as valerian, skullcap, lemon balm are good to calm the nerves. Also deep breathing exercises.

LOW AIR

I was very surprised that Carl Sagan had low air because he was so brilliant. I find that sometimes this information works health-wise and sometimes it works personality-wise. Maybe one is not necessarily the other. Because it certainly works health-wise and he died too young of cancer. And he compensated for the low air by becoming a great scientist. Astrologer Bob Marks feels that with low air in the chart every word you say is important or has meaning. You probably don't waste time in trivial discussions. Low air can have a difficulty in communicating. You don't always think things through. You can have poor judgment. And it can sometimes indicate a weak nervous system and a lack of a flow of bodily energies in the body. Also poor circulation. Poor movement. Movement therapies would help you. There can also be poor oxygenation, poor lung capacity. What was it we said about Peter Jenning? Peter Jennings had a lack of air which can be lung weakness. And there's a lack of flexibility in the body with low air. Too much earth is also a lack of flexibility and coordination. Do group work to help increase communication skills. Go dancing. Use incense as an air cure. Have pleasant smells around you. Nice sounds and agreeable scents in the air are cures for low air. A white noise machine can be a cure for low air also. Have fresh, circulating air around you. Engage in sports that promote agility such as golf which you can also play outdoors in fresh air. Wear sky blue colors and to stimulate brain activity there is a Chinese herb called gotu kola. And another one called fo ti. You can find a lot of these Chinese herbs at Pearl River on lower Broadway in New York City.

Audience: What about essential oils such as peppermint?

DC: You can use essential oils for nice smells. You sprinkle the oil on a heated light bulb in a lamp and the smell carries throughout your home.

Audience: What did you say about gotu kola?

DC: Gotu kola stimulates the brain and fo ti is sometimes referred to as the Chinese elixir of life. And of course wearing sky colors stimulates low air. Color therapy can be very useful, but it's not a subject that we discuss a lot. Apparently, it can help you with health problems. Remember you can use colors in decorating as well as in clothing.

WATER ELEMENT

When water is balanced in your chart, you are sensitive, caring, compassionate, loving, psychic and aware. So if water is emphasized in your chart you can be spiritual or creative, or you need to be emotionally involved in whatever you do.

EXCESS WATER

If you have too much water, such as Carl Sagan has a water emphasis, you are very receptive but you can be dependent on other people for your emotional fulfillment. You may also be very conservative. You are very attuned to emotions, symbols and the arts. You can be very defensive. Sagan sure was defensive when it came to astrology.

Water has strong ties to the past. With excess water you can be prone to depression and experience moodiness. You can avoid reality. Also, there can be a lack of boundaries when you have too much water. You need to learn to be more detached. Years ago there was a book called *Psychic Self-Defense* by Dion Fortune that was very popular. And it teaches you to put an invisible wall around yourself. And if you have a lot of water in your chart, you may not be ill, but the person next to you could be, so you start feeling ill. And if you are very watery and deal with sick people, you need to do something to protect yourself. You are like a psychic sponge picking up impressions and vibrations around you. It's like that old expression about people stealing your energy. You pick up energy because it is just drawn to you. So you have to put an invisible wall around yourself.

Too much water can cause phlegm. You can be over-weight, bloated, have swellings, mucous discharge. Ingrid Naiman, who has written a few medical astrology books, talks about how too much water causes waxy deposits in the body that build up and need to be melted. And she said that turmeric is a good heating spice to melt these deposits. I've been reading a lot about the helpful effects of turmeric in general. She said these waxy deposits can become toxic in the body. She also said that spices, saunas and hot baths can melt them. She considers these deposits as stagnant water that has hardened and needs to be melted and dried out or it will erode the other elements. These deposits will congest your body. Swedish bitters are helpful also. So with excess water you can be nauseous, bloated, have swellings, breast lumps, prostate swelling, lymphatic swelling. You have to be careful of cold, wet, sweet foods such as ice cream and watermelon when you have a lot of water. You are better off with foods that dry you such as popcorn or crackers. Foods that crumble or are brittle are good for excess water. They dry you out.

Sometimes I find this information so simplified. Wish that it would work. Mostly these are suggestions that can help balance your body. Wouldn't it be nice to eat crackers and get rid of some horrible health problem. I wish it were that easy. So we have to look at all this realistically. I believe that toxins build up over the years, and possibly if you are aware of a problem when you are young, you can prevent a lot of health problems when you a lot older. So use this information for preventative measures, not to cure a serious disease.

Audience: Do you think someone with a lot of water in their chart would naturally like to eat a lot of melon?

DC: They probably eat the things they shouldn't. Right.

Edgar Cayce said to eat melon alone. So if you're going to eat melon, don't eat it with a meal. Eat it alone. So maybe with some foods it's not that you shouldn't eat them, it's how and when you should eat them.

Audience: Is this for water people or for everyone?

DC: Everyone. He said that about melon in general. Take melon alone. He also said coffee was good for you. He said it was the milk in it that changed the acid content and caused it to become a problem and you should only drink it black. That's why I now only drink black coffee. It took me around two weeks to get used to it black, and now I don't like it with milk in it.

In terms of excess water, diuretic bitter tonics are good. Jane Ridder Patrick describes water as cold, wet and heavy and says it needs to be balanced by substances that are hot, dry and light. Dried fruits, heating spices like cayenne. You need exercise. You can also cure excess water with fire. Avoid a lot of oily foods. Avoid excess salt and foods such as bread that retain water. And find out what diuretic teas you like. And eat diuretic vegetables such as celery and asparagus.

LOW WATER

Scott Hamilton has weak water in his chart. It can indicate a difficulty showing emotions, being fearful, restless and hard to relax. You don't understand your feelings. You crave intimacy. You're afraid of emotional things at the same time. Water is the healing part of our bodies. Water heals and repairs tissues. So if you have low water, you can have poor healing. Also your body may not be smooth; you can become dehydrated, you may have brittle nails, stiff joints. You need rich, oily and moist herbs. Get an aquarium. Get one of those feng shui fountains. It was Doris Hebel who said that if water is low in your chart, float a fresh flower in a bowl of water and change the water every 2½ days when the Moon changes signs. Eat juicy fruits. Have squash and melons. Have a lot of soup. Eat puddings and custards. Learn how to project your feelings. How do you like this next one? Swim with the dolphins. Of course, I heard it was cruel to the dolphins. That's a way to increase the water element. Take baths. Take up painting. Creative activities bring in water. Nautical activities also. Doing healing work. Saunas. Hot baths. Avoid old food that has to be reheated. And medical astrologer Marcia Starck says that smoky quartz and black obsidian gemstones help to release old emotions.

Audience: Do you think transits and progressions have an effect on this information?

DC: I'll use progressed planets in that if you're getting some kind of difficult progression such as the progressed Sun coming to your Saturn, you may need more minerals. With a Uranus transit possibly more magnesium. I would use the progressions and also transits in terms of nutrition. You have to take each chart individually. You can't give a blanket answer for all charts. I look ahead to see the good and bad periods. I don't use the word "bad." I use the words "lack of vitality," "periods of stress," etc. Be careful of getting chilled, for example, during a Saturn transit. With Uranus Nodes, for example, I told someone to stay away from large stadiums or crowds. You could catch something during the flu season if you are having a Uranus Node or Node Uranus transit because Uranus Nodes indicates large groups of people among other meanings as well as sudden encounters.

Audience: I've seen people getting arrested on Uranus Node connections.

DC: Oh, really. Very interesting. I'd also look at aspects such as Neptune to Mars or Neptune to the Sun. I'd avoid large crowds with that combination also during the flu season, for example. If someone is really ill, when you examine their elements and modes, you have useful information to give them. Because many times there is some type of imbalance in a chart. You may tell the client they have a lack of water in their chart and give cures for low water. You can look at the charts of individuals with great imbalances. Dick Cavett experienced depression.

Kurt Cobain committed suicide. David Crosby had a liver transplant and is the type to "burn-out." And Howard Hughes was a case of a mental disorder; Peter Jennings died of lung cancer, Madeline Kahn died of ovarian cancer; Scott Hamilton had cancer. And Nancy Hastings also had cancer. It's unfortunate how many cases you find of cancer. It's really depressing.

Audience: Something I noticed when you were talking about the overages and the lacks; I was sort of going through clients' charts in my head and realizing that they didn't have the lack but they had the aspect to the angles.

DC: Yes, that's why you look at aspects to the angles as you may have an affliction to a fixed angle so therefore you might have a proneness to fixed type of problems.

Audience: Question on the planets and the aspects.

DC: Well, it's going to be the old rules of astrology. Some modern astrologers say, "Oh, we don't have malefics." Really? You don't see anybody getting ill anymore or having an accident or whatever.

Audience: I don't think it's the idea that the planets cause the problem, but that the planets reflect the problem.

DC: Right. The planets show where the problems lie. If you learn medical astrology, and you see a Mars Neptune affliction in a chart, then one cure is to build up the adrenals. Or build up the immune system. That's the positive way to use the information.

Audience: What is your interpretation of someone who has Venus square Saturn – they might have problems with their skin?

DC: Skin problems. Right.

Audience: Would you tell the client not to worry. That they might have some kind of rash but in time it will go away.

DC: I usually don't even talk about health when I do general readings because most people don't want to hear about it. I would probably talk about their relationships and financial issues with Saturn Venus. You know you will have testing in relationships, or creativity or money issues or the issue with Saturn Venus of how you value yourself. Issues of self-esteem. If I were doing a health reading, then I would mention Saturn Venus in connection with skin disorders or in a worst case scenario lowered kidney function. I do health as a separate reading. I wouldn't ignore someone getting a Saturn transit to their Sun in a general reading by saying that everything is going to be just fine. In that case I might mention vitality problems or it being a good time to see a dentist. I want to evaluate the whole chart. If they don't have any health problems, let's not give them any. And as to your comment about telling a client the rash will go away, it might. Again you don't want to be diagnosing or ignoring what could be the symptoms of a deeper problem. Always recommend they see a doctor for a medical problem. A person with a rash might be helped by a dermatologist or possibly a nutritionist depending on the cause.

Audience: And you don't know how it will manifest.

DC: Right. You know you're going to have a test with Saturn or be forced to deal with reality. You know you will have less vitality. You may feel overwhelmed, even discouraged. And you may need more rest. So you can talk like that to the client.

Audience: As well as looking at the elements, do you look to see how the ruler of the sixth house is aspected?

DC: In my opinion, the ruler of the sixth is more about how your daily routines affect your health. However, when the ruler of the sixth house is in hard aspect to the ruler of the Ascendant, that can indicate a health issue usually related to the sign on the cusp of the sixth house or the Ascendant as well as vitality problems.

ADDITIONAL REFERENCES

1   Hill, Judith, *Medical Astrology,* Stellium Press, Portland, OR, 2004

2. Starck, Marcia, *Healing with Astrology*, The Crossing Press, Freedom, CA, 1997

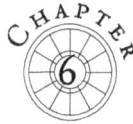

CHAPTER 6

HEALTH DISORDERS, ADDICTIONS AND STRESSORS IN THE NATAL CHART

This chapter focuses on recognizing the effects of addictions and stressors in undermining one's health. Significators of addictive behavior are given as well as information on identifying stressors in the natal chart.

Stressors and addictions can undermine health and your enjoyment of day-to-day life. You can't enjoy your love life or have a good day at work if you're sick. We can raise awareness and improve our health through the use of the natal chart. However, I don't think you can control genetics or a hereditary illness, which may be seen in the chart by an angular Pluto or sometimes by an afflicted Moon in the fourth or tenth house. Wanda Sellar discusses the use of the Nodes for hereditary diseases.[1] And as discussed in Chapter Four, some health problems can be traced back to the birth process. It can be a lack of oxygen or something that goes wrong with the delivery. Those things you can't do much about. In other respects, the natal chart can be useful in terms of health.

Audience: An angular Pluto to any planet?

DC: No, Pluto on an angle – specifically conjunct the Ascendant or MC, even the Descendant or the IC. As long as you use the word "angular."

Having an addiction can limit good health. What does it mean to be addicted to a food or substance? You are obsessed with something that you just can't get away from. You have to have it. If you look at a chart, those who have the toughest time breaking an addiction may have the Moon in a fixed sign. That is because the Moon has to do with habits and fixed signs can be resistant to change. The other Moon sign placements can break addictions easier so that's one thing to look for if your Moon is in a fixed sign or if you have a lot of fixed planets. However, the Moon in Scorpio, though a fixed sign, has a strong will once it decides to break an addiction.

What are some of the worst kinds of addictions? I believe they are either drugs, alcohol or food. I'm going to give you some significators for alcohol and drug addiction. Basically, the one planet that has the most to do with addiction is Neptune. And this is Neptune on an angle or Neptune in hard aspect to the Sun, Mercury or the Moon. That seems to show addiction. And Neptune is the planet that wants to break down barriers. And people who are addicted to drugs and alcohol find that these are substances that break down barriers. So, therefore, they have a sense of oneness with all. And that's the spiritual side of Neptune which when not manifesting in a positive way can express itself in drugs or alcohol or a need to escape reality. You can become addicted to TV also as well as the Internet. And I think the most difficult aspect in the chart is the Moon in a hard aspect to Neptune in terms of addiction. It's easy to delude yourself with a Moon Neptune aspect.

In my *Dictionary of Medical Astrology*[2] I listed the following combinations for Addiction:

Neptune Ascendant, Moon Neptune, Jupiter Neptune, Mars Neptune, Moon = Mars/Neptune.

As far as food addiction, the two signs that I have seen that have the most problems with compulsive eating are Taurus and Cancer. Or you might see a stellium in the second house, which is the natural house of Taurus or a stellium in the fourth house, which is the natural house of Cancer. I usually find it's problems in the sign of Taurus or Cancer, and I've also seen food addiction with hard aspects involving Moon Jupiter or Venus Jupiter.

Audience: What is a stellium?

DC: A stellium is four or more planets in one house or sign. Supposedly a true stellium needs to include the Sun or the Moon, but I don't necessarily agree. If you have four or more planets in one sign or house you've got a stellium which can be a strong emphasis in one part of the chart.

FOOD ADDICTION

How does a food addiction affect health? Because nutritionally, I think if you take care of yourself, I don't know if you will live longer but you can live healthier. We don't know when the clock in our bodies will stop, but why spend years of your life miserably sick or ill when if you are diligent about your health, you could be in reasonably good shape until your time comes, when hopefully, you will die of old age. That's my opinion of why you have to take care of yourself all your life, health-wise. So if you eat

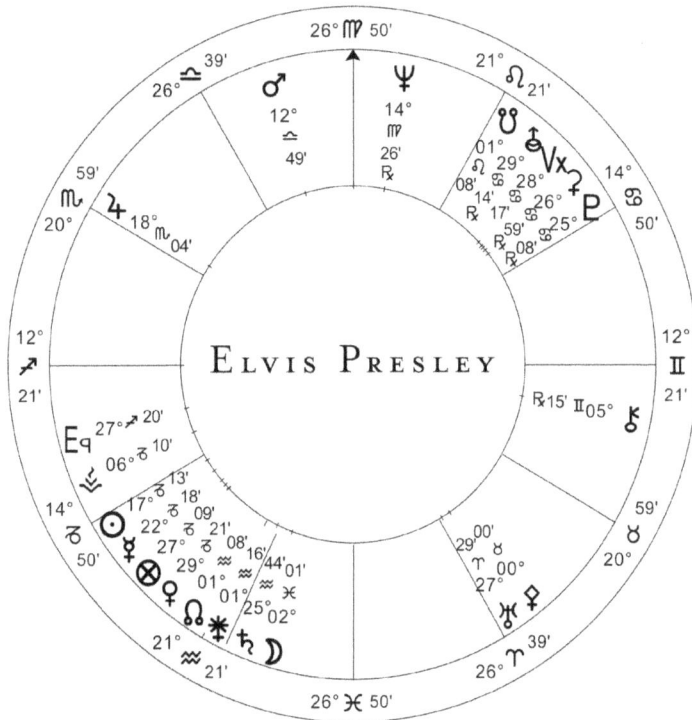

ELVIS PRESLEY

too much and you're obese, it affects your heart; it affects your whole body. And you are also prone to diabetes which can be a very difficult disease to live with. And you're just not healthy. You can have clogged arteries from too much fat. You probably don't have as much energy as you should either when you are carrying a lot of excess weight.

Elvis Presley is a good example of a person with food issues. He has some of the significators of weight gain in his chart. One is Jupiter in a water sign. He was a Sagittarius rising which also can indicate an expanded body or an indulgent personality. Sagittarius likes to do things in a big way and Elvis Presley tended to be extravagant in food, drink and drugs. He knew how to spend money also. He has three planets plus the North Node in his second house. There's that second house influence. Venus in the second intensifies the second house emphasis and the idea of indulgence. Venus is afflicted in his chart and that can indicate bad habits and gastrointestinal indiscretion. Stressful aspects to the Moon or Venus can also indicate food complexes. Both are stressed in his chart. Neptune elevated may indicate a need for escape or an addiction which in his case also included prescription drugs.

What is interesting is the asteroid Ceres in regard to food complexes. Demetria George in *Asteroid Goddesses* states that stressful aspects of Ceres to both the Moon and Venus can point to food complexes. Ceres is opposite Venus in Elvis Presley's chart. He also has Ceres conjunct Pluto. Martha Lang-Wescott mentions in *Mechanics of the Future* that combinations of Ceres Pluto can indicate food-related compulsions such as binge eating. She describes Ceres Pluto as an intense emotional crisis brought about through the loss or separation of loved ones. Elvis had a twin who died at birth. Lang-Wescott feels this can indicate a psychological complex that manifests in the diet. Elvis battled a weight problem most of his adult life and was known to go on food binges.

ALCOHOL AND DRUG ADDICTION

What is it with alcohol or drug addiction? Again, you always hear about people who have problems with their bodies from overuse of alcohol or drugs. So these can undermine your health.

Here's some information on alcoholism and drug addiction that I've come up with. Persons who are drug addicts or alcoholics come from families where one or more parent may have been an alcoholic. If you see a chart of someone who has Neptune conjunct the MC, they usually have an alcoholic parent. This would be true of Neptune conjunct the IC too. I'm giving you my experience. I've definitely seen Neptune on an angle with alcoholism. Some alcoholics are driven to alcohol through illness or depression. Some of them are just loners. They just can't form relationships with other people. Alcohol and drugs allow people to withdraw into their own world. They don't have to become a part of anything. Alcoholics and drug addicts may have a trace of impatience. They can't endure difficult circumstances. They have a lack of discipline. They are very angry at society.

There are astrological significators for addiction. Is there anyone who doesn't know what a significator is? There are astrological significators for everything. We are looking at significators of disease. In my first book *How to Give An Astrological Health Reading* I list significators for many diseases. You can just look at the specific significators along with the natal chart and if the person has a lot of significators for a particular illness, then they may have a proneness towards it. If they only have a couple of significators for a particular illness or disease, then it is usually not as much a problem. So when you're looking at significators, you want to see how many a person has for a particular problem.

SIGNIFICATORS OF ALCOHOL OR DRUG ADDICTION

The Sun or Moon weak in a chart, especially the Sun or Moon in fire or water, can indicate alcoholism or drug addiction. Mars in hard aspect to Neptune or a Pisces emphasis can have to do with drug addiction or alcoholism. When I say a Pisces emphasis what do I mean? A stellium in the 12th house or in the sign Pisces, or Neptune heavily afflicted as Neptune is the ruler of Pisces.

When you are a beginner this information sounds a little confusing. As you get into astrology, you find there is more than one way to see something in a chart. You have to look at all the ways too. Neptune angular or conjunct the Sun or the Moon has a lot to do with alcoholism or drug addiction. And, as I said earlier, the most difficult combination seems to be a hard aspect between the Moon and Neptune. Escapism into alcohol, drugs, food, even a fantasy world which is not part of this chapter, as I don't think fantasizing affects your health as much as drinking or doing drugs, but Moon Neptune can be a very difficult aspect to overcome.

Saturn Neptune combinations also show up in the charts of alcoholics or drug addicts. Also Jupiter Neptune, and you know why Jupiter Neptune is interesting? Jupiter rules Sagittarius, which rules the liver, and you know alcoholics can have problems with the liver. And Neptune also can be involved with the pancreas (ruler of Pisces opposite Virgo, the pancreas, on the mutable cross), and there can be problems with these organs when you drink too much. That's your Jupiter Neptune aspect.

Venus Neptune also for alcoholism and that can have to do with food too. Venus Neptune and Moon Jupiter are weight gain significators along with the signs Taurus and Cancer. And Venus Neptune, Mars Neptune and Mercury Neptune combinations are also associated with drugs and alcohol. And again, it keeps coming back to Neptune. Sun Neptune can describe an alcoholic father, because the Sun is supposed to represent the father in the chart. So you may find Sun Neptune in hard aspect or Neptune conjunct the MC that indicates the father was an alcoholic. It could be the mother too or an alcoholic family background.

Now here's an interesting one. Drugs are against the law. But alcohol is legal. Pluto rules the underworld. So you may find an angular Pluto or Pluto aspecting the Sun or the Moon showing up in the charts of drug addicts as opposed to alcoholics. You know when Pluto was discovered it was around the time of Prohibition and the rise of organized crime. So that's its connection to the underworld or the criminal element in society.

Audience: Question about hard aspects.

DC: When I say hard aspects I'm literally talking about any hard aspect, although I would say the square and opposition are the strongest but also the sesquiquadrate and semisquare along with other indications are strong. That's why I said, when you're looking at significators, if you just see one indication, such as someone who has a difficult Sun Neptune aspect in their chart, don't assume the person is an alcoholic, but if the chart also has a difficult Mars Neptune combination, and it was connected with the angular houses along with other indications, then you might say there is a tendency to addiction to drugs or alcohol.

Audience: What about the conjunction?

DC: I don't think the conjunction is as difficult as the square aspect as far as between malefics. I believe a difficult conjunction can undermine the sign or signs ruled which is a whole other topic. I don't think that conjunctions between malefics are as difficult as the square or opposition. The square is just like the old traditional books – very difficult. Moon square Neptune is a lot more difficult than the Moon conjunct Neptune not that I don't think the Moon Neptune conjunction isn't also difficult.

Audience: What about the trine?

DC: Some astrologers will say that a lot of trines make life too easy for you so you will start drinking if you have a Moon trine Neptune. I don't have enough charts to comment on this. I still like to go with the idea that malefics and hard aspects are difficult and good aspects are helpful. Because when is anything good going to happen to us if we are going to call trines bad. I've heard that with the Grand Trine that life is too easy; there's no struggle, and I've heard stories of bank robbers with Grand Trines – looking for a quick way to get money. You also know that Grand Trines can be very protective. So I'm going to stick to traditional astrology, hard aspects are difficult; easier aspects are easier to deal with.

Sometimes Jupiter connected with the Sun, Moon or another planet has to do with excess. So you can get into drugs or alcohol that way.

Another example of an addictive personality is Eric Clapton. He has overcome both a drug and alcohol addiction. He has the Moon in a fixed sign – Scorpio but

again a sign with the ability to break an addiction. He has
Neptune opposed to his Sun. He has a quincunx between
Mars and Neptune that could indicate an on/again off/
again involvement with drugs and alcohol. However, his
Mars is in Pisces and that intensifies the Mars-Neptune
aspect. Mars in Pisces can be another indication of addiction to drugs or alcohol. I mentioned that alcoholics and
drug addicts can be impatient. He is an Aries, a normally
impatient sign and his ruler Mars is square Uranus. If you
recall in Chapter Four (Mental Aberrations in the Chart) I
mentioned Dr. William Davidson's theory that alcoholics
drink due to a spasm condition in their body that can be
indicated by a hard aspect between Mars and Uranus. As

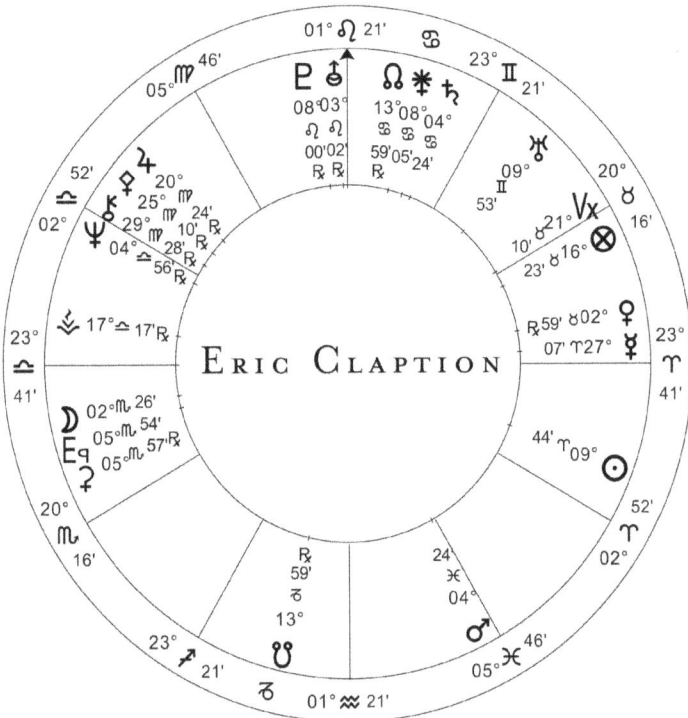

ERIC CLAPTON

mentioned the Sun or Moon weak in a chart, especially the Sun or Moon in fire or water, along with other indicators can indicate alcoholism or drug addiction. He has the Sun in Aries (fire) and the Moon in Scorpio (water) in fall. He has Saturn square Neptune, another significator of alcohol or drug addiction as well as Venus in hard aspect to Neptune..

A similarity to Elvis Presley's chart is that both have Ceres opposite Venus. And Ceres is square Pluto in Clapton's chart and conjunct Pluto in Presley's chart. As Wescott states Ceres Pluto is an intense emotional crisis brought about through the loss or separation of loved ones.

As stated in Wikipedia:

"Clapton grew up with his grandmother, Rose, and her second husband Jack, believing they were his parents and that his mother was his older sister."

I mentioned an angular Pluto showing up in the charts of drug addicts. Pluto is elevated in the 10th house in Eric Clapton's chart.

The preceding is what I would look for as far as alcoholism, drug abuse and food as an addiction or a compulsive trait in your life that is hard to break and which can ultimately undermine your health.

Audience: You say drugs or alcohol a lot. And sometimes you put food in there.

DC: At the beginning I said I was describing three things we can be addicted to that undermine our health – drugs, alcohol and food.

Audience: I don't agree with food since you have to eat.

DC: I was saying you could have a food addiction if the signs Taurus or Cancer are emphasized. Then food becomes addictive. If you weigh 300 pounds, you are stressing your heart and you're undermining your health.

Audience: Yes, I know that.

DC: You don't think food can be an addiction?

Audience: No, I do. I just think it's different than drugs or alcohol.

DC: Well, food addiction can undermine your health as well as addiction to drugs or alcohol. Obviously, persons addicted to drugs or alcohol can be more of a danger to society than someone with a food addiction.

I think that people can be addicted to television too or even the Internet, but I wouldn't say those addictions undermine your health. Maybe it undermines your spine or increases the size of your backside. And those are sedentary habits. I'm basically trying to discuss what can undermine our health that can shorten our lives.

Audience: At first you said your Moon sign. I would think that if you have your Moon in Scorpio you have a stronger will to break a habit.

DC: I agree as I have a Scorpio Moon. I still think you have to get by the rigid and extremist part of a Scorpio Moon first. Having a Scorpio Moon I know what it's like. I was able to stop smoking, which is another addiction. And smoking is an addiction that obviously undermines your health, and it can be shown by excess mutability in the chart. Giving up cigarettes took a lot of will. It still was hard to break the smoking habit.

Possibly the Scorpio Moon doesn't go back to smoking. Because once I stopped, I stopped. You know you hear people have stopped smoking for ten years, and then they go back to a pack a day. Maybe the Scorpio Moon gives the will to stay away from cigarettes once you quit. It's still difficult. It's still a fixed Moon. You still have rigid habits or bad habits that can be hard to break.

STRESS AND HEALTH

The other topic I wanted to discuss is stress itself which most health professionals believe contributes to poor health and disease. How well you handle stress can sometimes determine how healthy you are. To a certain extent I think that if you can't handle stress, it can undermine your health. Some health practitioners think that conditions such as ulcers, arthritis, heart disease and cancer are linked to the type of personality you have and how you handle stress. And when you can deal appropriately with stress, then your health improves.

Now what is stress? It is any stimulus that affects your body. Even if it's a positive stimulus, it can still be stressful. Have you seen those studies that list 100 things that can happen to you in one year and how the people who checked the most events on the list died or experienced a serious health problem? And some of the events were good, such as getting married and getting engaged. They had on the list such things as death of a parent, loss of a job, moving, husband died, etc. and the more points you had, the more stress you had in one year and the sicker you became to the point that some people died because they had so much stress in one year. And again, it doesn't have to be bad stress. It doesn't matter what causes the stress; it's how you handle it.

PREDICTING PERIODS OF STRESS

Mars in your chart may show how you handle stress. Mars is fight, fright, or flight. Stress is cumulative; it accumulates to the point where you just flip out one day from the buildup so you have to learn how to handle it. And you may know when you will have stress by using predictive techniques. Periods of stress can be seen astrologically by squares, oppositions, quincunxes, semisquares or sesquiquadrates by outer planets to personal points. If you saw Uranus by transit to your Sun, don't you think you might be having a stressful time? Or to your Moon? So that's when you might see periods of stress.

I want to refer you back to Chapter Five: "Rebalancing with the Elements and the Modes" and the discussion of Cardinal, Fixed and Mutable personalities. Basically cardinal types need to learn how to relax, fixed types need to learn to be more adaptable and flexible, and mutable types need to learn how to focus their attention and avoid negative thinking.

In terms of stress in relation to the houses, I would say that there are three houses in the chart that deal with the ability to handle stress. That would be the first house, the third house and the sixth house. If you have a lot of difficult planetary aspects involving the first house, you may get stressed out easily. Or you have problems in handling stress. The third house is a mental house and an emphasis of planets in that house can indicate you experience anxiety or mental exhaustion. Eileen Nauman[3] calls third house problems the "disease of peopling." You may always be surrounded by a lot of people when you have a third house emphasis or just being surrounded by a lot of people causes you stress, and you just need to get away and be by yourself. You're just making yourself nervous and irritable which puts a strain on the nervous system that in turn undermines your health. And the sixth house is similar as many times with a sixth house emphasis, you can have trouble handling stress. Or you are a workaholic which puts a strain on the physical body. Or possibly you have a problem in dealing with co-workers which can also be stressful. The sixth house can refer to functional disorders that disrupt your daily routines or are caused by a disruption in your daily routines.

Mars in the first can describe people who don't know when to stop; they don't know their own limits. I have mentioned earlier in the book the case of a man with Lou Gehrig's disease who I know was a person who said he never slowed down. And obviously there are significators that show Lou Gehrig's disease, but I thought it was interesting that he was a person who did put a lot of stress on his body. You can lower your immune system through stress. The parts of your chart that show weakness or proneness to disease are where you might get ill, I believe, if you become totally stressed out and you don't take care of yourself. However, if you see certain weaknesses in the chart, but you take care of yourself you should just experience functional problems. If you don't take care of yourself, and you burn out and you never rest, such as Mars in the first type people, your body suddenly can't take the strain anymore and the weaknesses in the chart may then manifest as disease. That is my belief about health and medical astrology and how you can use it to help you. So a difficulty in dealing with stress can be shown by malefics in the first, third or sixth house or to the rulers of those houses. I have also found that persons with an angular Uranus, especially elevated, may have a difficulty in dealing with stress.

Look at the Sun for vitality. And look at the Sun for your will. If you have a weak will, I don't think you handle stress well because you could have an inferiority complex and you can experience psychological problems. So a strong, well-aspected Sun will give you a stronger personality and stronger vitality and the ability to stand up for yourself. And if you have a weak Sun, build it up health wise. You can do this by getting more sunlight and exercising more. Do activities that empower you to build up your Sun. Seek psychological help if necessary. Review Stephen Arroyo's[4] advice from Chapter Five where you use the element of your sun sign to help rejuvenate you. Whatever your sun sign is, whatever element it is in can help rejuvenate you. And people tend to forget that simple advice; use your Sun sign if you forget everything else.

Audience: Do you take into account the ruler of the sixth?

DC: As previously mentioned, when the ruler of the sixth is in hard aspect with the Ascendant or the ruler of the Ascendant that can indicate a potential health problem according to the sign on the Ascendant.

This is a complex subject and it takes years to learn and understand. I've been studying medical astrology for years and it's just starting to come together for me. Lecturing and writing on medical astrology has helped me because I've had to go into my notes and learn things to teach to the audience or write about. And that's the best way to learn. Just practice on charts. Find a person with a particular disease and take the chart and see if you can find the indications. You have to go backwards. Don't try to diagnose people. You can't do that.

1   Sellar, Wanda, *Introduction to Medical Astrology,* The Wessex Astrologer, Bournemouth, England, 2008.

2   Cramer, Diane, *Dictionary of Medical Astrology,* AFA, Tempe, AZ, 2003.

3   Nauman, Eileen: *The American Book Of Nutrition & Medical Astrology,* Astro Computing Services, San Diego, CA, 1982.

4   Arroyo, Stephen, *Astrology, Psychology and the Four Elements,* CRCS Publications, Davis, California, 1975.

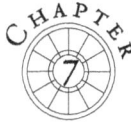

CHAPTER 7

RECOGNIZING AND TREATING WORKPLACE STRESS

This chapter focuses on the effects of stress in relation to the workplace. The needs of each sign in relation to work satisfaction are given. Acid-alkaline imbalance is discussed. Also included is useful information on the transits of Saturn through Pluto in the vocational houses – 2, 6 and 10 and a discussion of the role of the inner transits in terms of stress. Information on the use of the planets for treatment is included.

Medical astrology can help you deal with stress in the workplace by an understanding of your personal sun sign. I feel that if you don't fulfill your sun sign, you are going to incur stress. That's a simplistic way of looking at the issue, but I'm going to discuss what each sign needs in terms of satisfaction to avoid stress in the workplace.

Here is a definition of stress that I found on Dictionary.com.

> a mentally or emotionally disrupting condition occurring in response to adverse external influences and capable of affecting physical health usually characterized by increased heart rate, a rise in blood pressure, muscular tension, irritability and depression. A stimulus or circumstance causing such a condition. A state of extreme difficulty, pressure or strain.

I'll also be discussing the acid/alkaline balance in the body and its role in disease. It's becoming a more popular topic in that being too acidic can lead to disease. I want to point out to you that when we're talking about acidity to think of acid rain. Acid is destructive to the environment as well as to our bodies. Geocities.com says, "Acid rain is an extremely destructive form of pollution, and the environment suffers from its effects. Forests, trees, lakes, animals, and plants suffer from acid rain." So what do you think too much acid is doing to your body? It can harm us also. This is slightly simplistic, but not really. The more acidic you are, the more you are undermining your health. A combination of wrong eating and stress increases acid in the body. And if you are in the workplace having a bad day, you become more acidic. So that's why I'm going to include acid/alkaline information. Because, apparently, at a certain point, when you are really overstressed, the body can no longer eliminate acid so what happens is that the acid goes into your joints, tissues and bones and that's the beginning of disease. So I'll give you some of the information I've gleaned from two books that I've been studying.

Toxins causes stress. Noise causes stress. Anger causes stress. I arbitrarily picked 12 people using the 12 signs of the zodiac so that we could look at each one briefly to see how they fulfill their sun sign. Fulfilling your sun sign helps reduce stress. And I also have information on transits going through the houses of work that can cause stress – houses 2, 6 and 10.

You want your body to be neither too acidic nor too alkaline. So the main thing that you want to do to live a healthy life is use the ratio 80/20 – 80% alkaline-forming food, 20% acid-forming food. And it's almost impossible to eat that way because the foods we love tend to be more acidic. If you find that you are very acidic, if you can use the 80/20 formula, you can bring your body back into balance. So the question is how do you determine your acid/alkaline balance. And the two books I read have different opinions. *The Acid/Alkaline Diet*[1] has a whole chapter on testing your urine using litmus paper. And it's a lot of work and I don't know if anyone would really want to do that every day. The other book, *Alkalize or Die*[2], has a list of stressors. In fact the author has an acid symptom checklist, and when you're done evaluating your answers, you can then determine if you're too acidic. And he claims you can't use the litmus paper as your body keeps changing all day long. See the following website for more information on acid/alkaline imbalance in the body and the conditions that can develop from mild acidity. Note also the following information on pH taken from this site:

http://www.naturalhealthschool.com/acid-alkaline.html

> pH (potential of hydrogen) is a measure of the acidity or alkalinity of a solution. It is measured on a scale of 0 to 14—the lower the pH the more acidic the solution, the higher the pH the more alkaline (or base) the solution. When a solution is neither acid nor alkaline it has a pH of 7 which is neutral.

> Water is the most abundant compound in the human body, comprising 70% of the body. The body has an acid-alkaline (or acid-base) ratio called the pH which is a balance between positively charged ions (acid-forming) and negatively charged ions (alkaline-forming.) The body continually strives to balance pH. When this balance is compromised many problems can occur.

Astrologically, in terms of balance in the body, I have found that anyone who has Saturn in the cardinal signs, especially Saturn in Cancer, can have a problem with acid/alkaline balance and also with producing enough hydrochloric acid to assimilate nutrients in the body. Our bodies are so finely tuned that the smallest imbalance can lead to illness.

An unbalanced pH in the body tends toward acidity. You can look at the sign Libra which rules the kidneys for acid/alkaline imbalance in the body. From Wikipedia: "They (the kidneys) are part of the urinary system, but have several secondary functions concerned with homeostatic functions. These include the regulation of electrolytes, acid-base balance, and blood pressure." Afflictions involving the sign Libra or its ruler Venus can indicate imbalance in the body.

The planet of alkalinity is Saturn and the planet of acidity is Mars. So you're trying to find a fine balance between Mars and Saturn also. And you could also see if you're more acidic or alkaline by seeing which is stronger in your chart – Mars or Saturn. You can be too alkaline too. That's not good either. Sun Mars problems seem to indicate acidity in the body. Mars Saturn in hard aspect can cause the acid/alkaline balance to be off. Mars rules acidity; Saturn rules alkalinity. Mars in Cancer is a problem just like Saturn in Cancer is a problem. All of these placements can lead to an imbalance in the body. That's what it really amounts to – noting imbalances. And Mars in a cardinal sign can be acidic.

You're supposed to have a 20%/80% ratio of acid to alkaline. And the strongly acid foods are meat, fish and soft drinks. The mild acid foods are grains, legumes and nuts. The mild alkaline foods are fruits, vegetables, berries and dairy. The strongly alkaline foods are green leafy vegetables, broccoli and spinach. You can supplement your diet with alkaline minerals. There are lists in the backs of the source books and on the website healingdaily.com of companies that sell alkaline minerals, as you can improve yourself by just taking minerals that help alkalize you. If you have a health problem, you might be able to start improving your health just by following this 80/20 ratio or by taking food enzymes or green food supplements. Before you make extreme changes in your diet, you should see a doctor or nutritionist.

There's also an alkalizing lifestyle where you can change the way you live and improve your way of life. I'll just give you a couple of examples taken from *The Acid/Alkaline Diet*[1]. A sedentary lifestyle is acidifying. An active one is alkalizing. Taking the elevator is acidifying. Taking the stairs is alkalizing. You travel by car; it is acidifying. You travel by foot as much as possible, it alkalizes you. Passive hobbies acidify and active leisure pursuits alkalize. If you are outdoors a lot it helps you; if you are indoors a lot it doesn't. Being stressed obviously acidifies you. Taking your time alkalizes you. Being restless, always short on time is very acidifying. Being relaxed and organized is very alkalizing. Restless sleep and insomnia is acidifying. Sleeping soundly is alkalizing.

Need I say more. Pessimistic vs. optimistic. Loses temper easily; irritable. Think of Moon Mars – a very acidifying combination. Serene vs. impatient. Aggressive, envious and jealous vs. confident and tranquil. So you can look at your chart in terms of those characteristics and your own lifestyle and in the foods you eat. There are ways to become more alkaline without even having to change your diet. It's like a mindset. It's learning to take everything in stride and not overreacting which is not easy if you have a hard Moon Uranus or Moon Mars aspect in your chart.

As mentioned, I arbitrarily picked 12 people to represent each sign. I'll discuss what each sign needs in terms of vocation and then we'll look at the individual charts.

First are the requirements of each element.

Fire signs like risk, excitement and danger. Those are attributes that could cause stress to an earth sign. So again, to fulfill your sun sign if it's in fire you like challenge and conflict. You thrive on it. And if you have a lot of excess adrenaline, you can do mountain climbing; you can go to the health club. You can go rollerblading. Fire needs to have a way to burn off excess energy, but fiery types still thrive on excitement.

All earth signs need stability. They find a lot of change stressful. So if you are an earth sign you need job security and tend to dislike frequent job changes. You are going to stick with one thing or have stress.

Air signs have to be in a sociable environment or job. And there's a social or intellectual element involved. You have to use your intellect if you are an air sign. And you need to be able to communicate in some way.

Water signs need to be emotionally involved in whatever they do. They're good at handling other people's emotional problems. I think water signs need to be in a creative environment also. We'll talk about each water sign specifically.

Now this is Sun sign astrology but you could use the information for any emphasis in the chart such as a strong Aries, for example, or you could use it for a stellium in a sign.

ARIES

Let's look at Hugh Heffner's chart, an example of an Aries. Aries has a tendency to overdo it, which leads to acidity. Even if you are the type of person who works out at the

25° Ⅱ 10'

29° ♋ 04'

⚷ ☊ ♇ ♀ ⚸
24° 21° 12° 05° 00°
♋ ♋ ♋ ♋
17° 16' 37' 31' 57'
S ℞

21° ♉ 29'

41'
♃
⊗ 13°
♆ 20° ♌ 32'
♌ 22° ♌ 11'
29° ♌ 08' ℞

♂ 27° 21° ♈ 20'
20° ♈
18' ♈ 19° ☉

25°
♍ Eq 24° ♍ 16'
52'

H U G H   H E F F N E R

℞ 15' ♈ 03' ☿
46' ♓ 26° ♅
25°
♓
52'
58' ♓ 18°
36' ♓ 13° Vx
☽

21°
♎ 20'

℞ 06'
♏ 25°

℞ 16'
♐ 21°

21'
45' ♒ 03°
40' ♒
48' ♒ 22°
♒ 20°
12° ♒ 29°
♃
♀ 41'
✳
♂

21°
♏ 29'
♄

☋ 04'
29° ♐

25° ♐ 10'

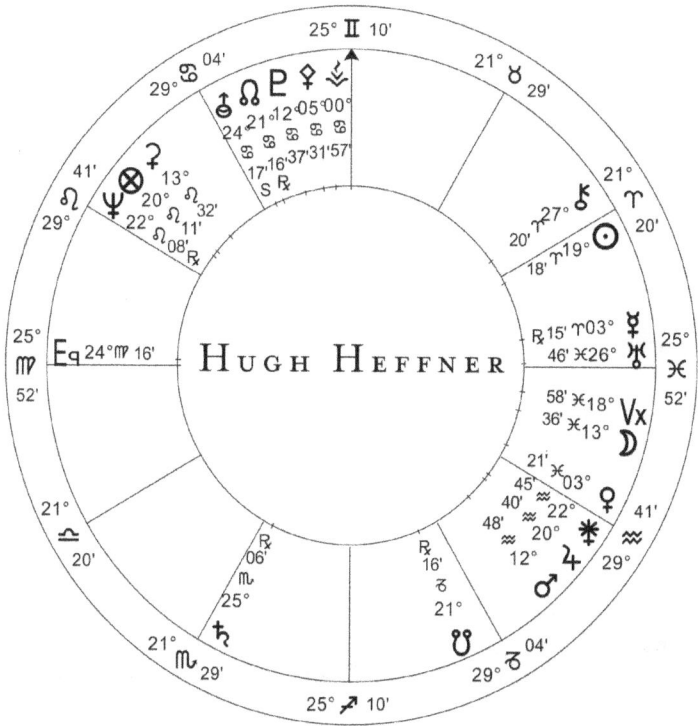

gym constantly, it's not healthy. You can be pushing your body too hard. And Aries can be like that. And Aries is very immature and can quit a job when feeling pressured. In terms of work, Aries doesn't like being talked down to. Aries needs independent action at work, doesn't like taking orders and needs autonomy. So in order to fulfill your sun sign if you are an Aries, you have to be in charge or you feel stressed. So if you take a job and people are ordering you around or you do not have independent action and your Sun is in Aries, you can experience a great deal of stress. You have to find an area of life where authority or autonomy is possible.

Let's look at Hugh Heffner. I tried to find business people and it was interesting when I got to Cancer how many rich and famous people had their Sun in Cancer. Very wealthy people. Hugh Heffner is an Aries. Aries can be the first at something. I thought it was humorous in a way. I don't know if you ever heard this about Pluto, but I once learned that Pluto is the first time you do something and the last time you do something. First and lasts. And Hugh Heffner was one of the first publishers of flesh magazines involving women. "Playboy." And look at Pluto elevated in his 10th house. Pluto rules sex. And then I had a laugh. What's a good way to relieve stress with Pluto? Think of Hugh Heffner at the Playboy mansion and you've got a nice stress reliever there. Later I want to talk about planets in high stress and what they mean also. How does he reduce stress in a Plutonian way? The main thing is that he is an Aries; he was one of the first to start something; he is an entrepreneur. And he is in charge and he fulfills his sun sign. And notice he has an angular Uranus. That will indicate something different about the life. And how about his unusual life style and love affairs and marriage with Uranus in the seventh. He has both Pluto and Uranus angular in his chart. When I'm trying to simplify something, I just look at the angles of the chart or the angular houses. And he was a first at something and he certainly has a unique lifestyle. So I thought he was a good example of an Aries.

TAURUS

Now, what does Taurus need? We are going to look at Liberace who is a perfect example of enjoying opulence and luxury – a Taurean trait. Taurus doesn't do well in a fast-paced, unpredictable work environment. Taurus likes to take things slowly and do things their own way. They like to be in a comfortable atmosphere. They have a tendency to be too sedentary. Remember we just saw that being too sedentary contributes to acidity. So you have to be careful about that. Taurus needs an outlet. They need to do something involving bodywork or something physical.

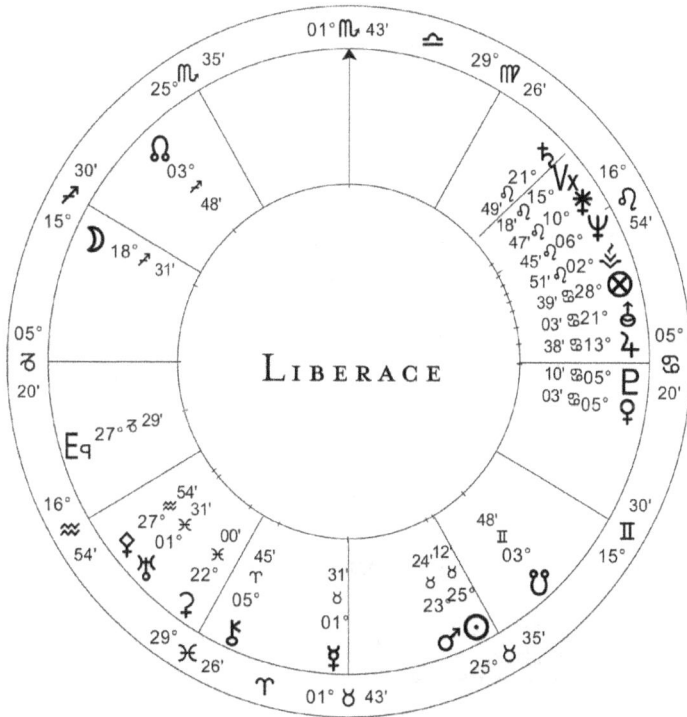

LIBERACE

Taurus is a sign that likes its leisure time. I don't think Taurus would do well working all day with no breaks. And they don't like jobs with overtime. They are very good at physical work. They need intimacy, regular meals and physical contact. Think of earth as something physical. A comfy chair at the office could make all the difference in the world. Otherwise stress. This is what we're trying to see. If you don't fulfill your sign work-wise, what could be the result?

Now look at Liberace. Think of luxury and he was a perfect example with all the candles, the glitter, the gold during his performances. I noticed that his Sun was on Algol, 25 Taurus, and he did die of AIDS. Algol is a malefic fixed star. And he does have a Venus Pluto conjunction on the Descendant. That could also describe a sexual disease. Also, when you're looking at a chart, look at the most elevated planet, which in this case is Saturn. He had to have a lot of discipline also to be an entertainer with all the work it took. Or it could indicate the fact that he ended up with health problems – you could look at Saturn that way also. Mercury is also angular conjunct the 4th house cusp opposite the MC, and he was an entertainer. I noticed Algol when I was first looking at the chart. He was also quite energetic and an excellent piano player which could be shown by the Sun Mars conjunction. The Sun Mars could also mean he was too acidic. There's a clue.

Audience: And it's square Saturn.

DC: Right. That creates more of an imbalance. I think he personifies Taurus if nothing else.

GEMINI

Donald Trump is a Gemini. Isn't he everywhere? He's on
television; he's on ads; he's on Saturday Night Live. He's
certainly all over the place. Gemini obviously needs a lot
of variety in work. And they need jobs that have flexibility
or involve dexterity. And sometimes they can be very non-
committal so any job that requires a lot of passion or com-
mitment is not really good for Gemini as they're always
off to the next thing. They experience insomnia sometimes
and that contributes to stress. Insomnia is a contributor to
stress no matter what your sign is. Gemini needs to learn
how to finish projects once they start them.

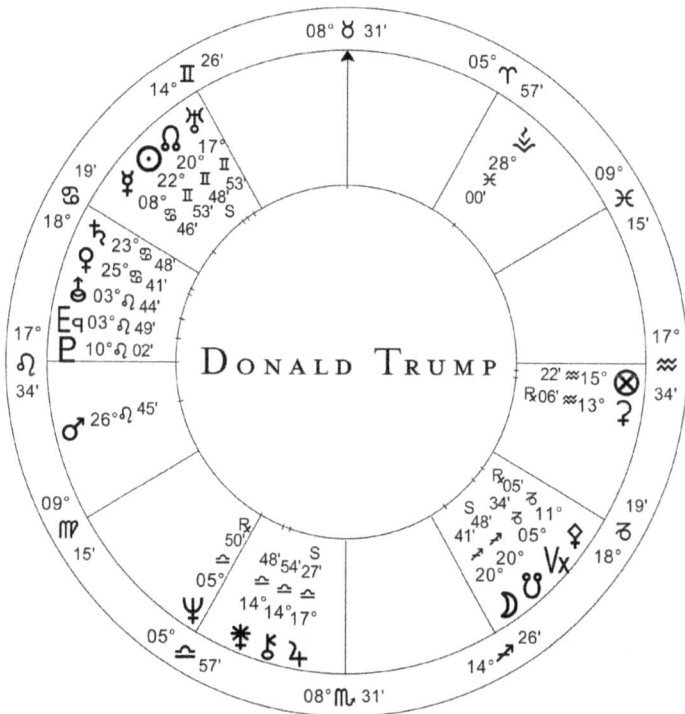

193

They enjoy books and any kind of playful exercise is good for Gemini. The main thing is having a job that involves variety.

Now, if we look at Donald Trump we see he has Mars in the first house. Obviously, you're not going to just take someone's Sun sign and give an interpretation because his Sun is near the Nodes and Uranus so we have a unique individual right there who makes important connections. And Uranus is his most elevated planet. He is probably extremely hyper. You know he's out practically every night of the week. He says he'd like to stay home, but I doubt it. Look at how hyper this chart is: Mars in the first house, Uranus elevated conjunct the Sun and Pluto applying to the Ascendant. I wouldn't give Pluto too much first house influence as it's more in the 12th house, but it is rising above the Ascendant. He just has to do things that require diversity and energy. I would say once you get past the sun sign, you can go into more detail to learn about the profession as certainly Taurus at the top of his chart shows his desire to acquire things in life. You get more information as you study the MC's. And I was just noticing that Hugh Heffner has Gemini on the MC, which can be magazines. So that's interesting.

Audience: What do you do with Transpluto?

DC: Oh, I put in Transpluto because it's a super Pluto. Where Pluto is supposed to be a higher octave of Mars, Transpluto is a higher octave of Pluto. And Eleanor Kimmell, the cosmobiologist, uses Transpluto and I started using it after hearing her talk about it in lectures and discussing it in her books. I have my two famous cases of Transpluto. I wish I had more, but I haven't had time to investigate it. The moment that Dale Earnhardt, the famous race car driver, died in Daytona Beach in 2001, Transpluto was on the Ascendant of the event chart. And if you look at the New Moon chart before 9/11, the New Moon was conjunct Transpluto. And I use New Moon charts to predict from month to month, even more than lunar returns. I find that the New Moon chart gives me more information. So those are two cases of Transpluto. They are pretty potent examples. And one medical astrologer, Eileen Nauman, says that if you have Transpluto rising in your chart it indicates hypoglycemia. I just throw it in to observe. Everyone has something they throw into a chart. That's mine. I think there's something to it.

CANCER

Cancer needs emotional work and job security. They don't like to be criticized. They can be very moody. And Cancer can stress out co-workers with their moods. Now some signs stress out other people because they are impossible to be around. Cancer can be that way sometimes. A major thing with Cancer seems to be food issues. So malnutrition is going to contribute to stress also. Or they eat to get over stress causing weight gain. It depends on what you're eating, but eating a lot of junk food can make you more acidic. So Cancer needs to have emotional security and emotional ties and domestic security. And certainly Leona Helmsley had domestic security. Do your remember that she went to jail? She was called the "Queen of Mean." I thought it was interesting that her Sun is in the 12th house and she ended up in jail. The 12th house can be a house of confinement. And she was also known for her

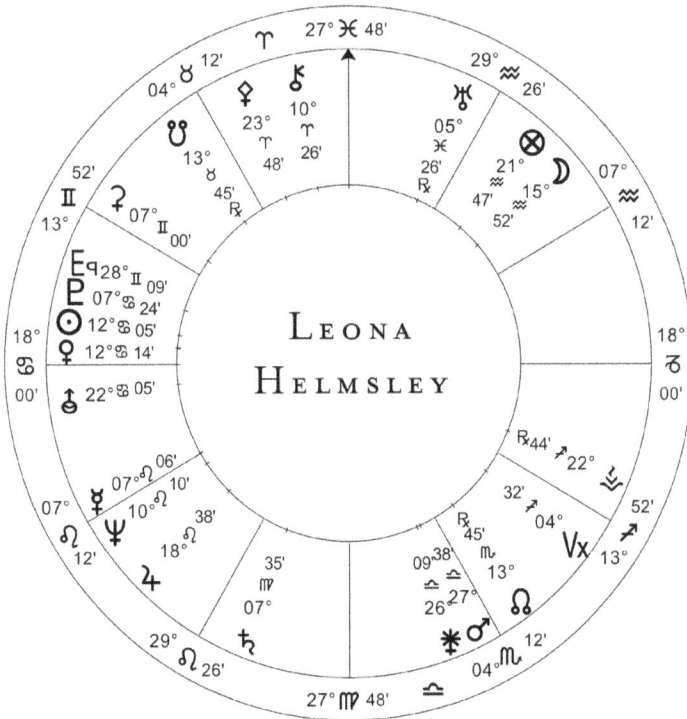

moods. She acquired property by marrying into it. With Capricorn on the 7th, she was looking for status through marriage. She is an example of some of the worst of Cancer and some of the best from what has been written about her.

LEO

Leo people need some kind of self-importance and a job that leaves time for recreation. Leo likes to have a good time. They don't like working for other people or dealing

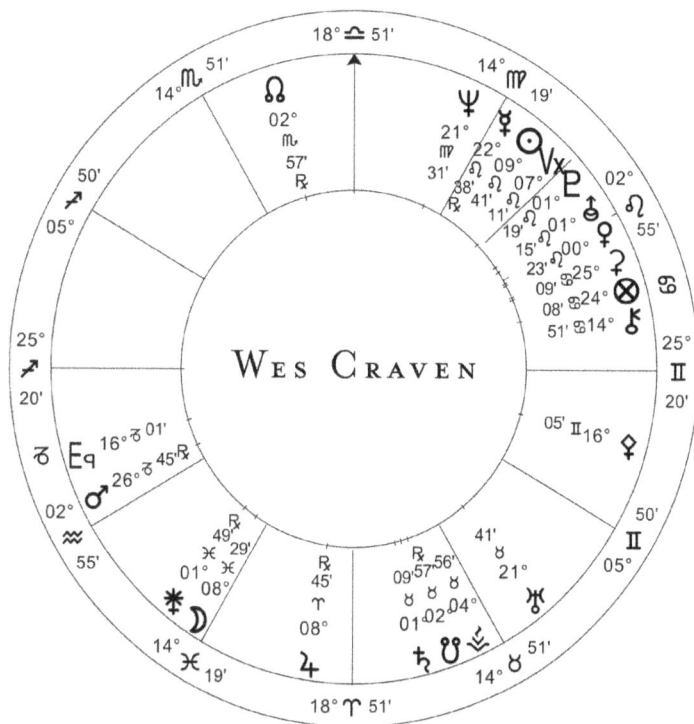

WES CRAVEN

with petty details. They don't like routine. They want to make a splash. And they tend to think they are always right. Leo can be dramatic and needs to express themselves in some way. They also like to gamble and take chances. And I thought Wes Craven was a good example. He's into filmmaking. He has Neptune elevated at the top of his chart. Neptune is associated with film or anything make-believe. I think Neptune elevated in the chart or in the 10th house combined with the sign Leo has a lot to do with the theater. Anything with Neptune can be film or glamour or even scandal. He's made a lot of horror movies. He has a Mars Pluto opposition out of sign, but he does have the opposition. So that aspect may represent the kind of movies he makes as Mars Pluto can be a violent combination. He's also an example of a creative person who found his niche in the theater. That's a good example of a Leo.

VIRGO

Jimmy Connors will be our Virgo example. And Virgo has to work. Virgo is not going to be happy sitting around doing nothing. If Virgo has a job where they're not doing much of anything, they will become stressed. They can also become workaholics working double shifts, or they overdo it and don't know how to play so they make themselves more acidic that way. They need to feel useful. And they need tasks. And they also have to have control over their diet. Cancer also needs a communicative environment. Like Cancer they can have extremes in their diet.

Now Jimmy Connors does not look like a typical Virgo in the way we just described, but in order to become a top tennis player you have to hone your skills. And Virgo is very good at any kind of skill. And then I noticed that his Mars closely trines his MC. If you ever want to see success with money in a chart, if the ruler of the 10th is in the 2nd, or vice versa, you should be able to earn a good living. In Connor's case it was a close trine from 2 to 10. And he makes a living in a Martian way with a tennis racket. Mars is a physical planet. The chart will give you information, but it won't always be so obvious. As a Virgo, we know he became an expert in his field and with the

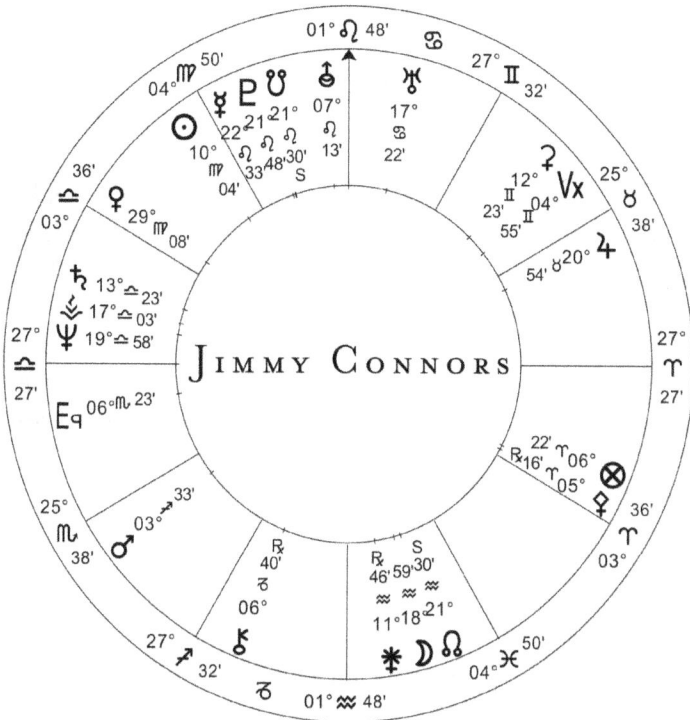

Leo MC he is famous in a theatrical way with tennis. He is a Virgo, and he had to have a skill that he developed which brought him to the top of his profession.

LIBRA

Johnny Carson ("The Tonight Show") is an example of a Libra. Certainly, he was a great socializer. Not necessarily a socializer on a one-to-one basis but everyone knew of him. He was great at talking with his guests. Also Libra has to have nice surroundings. Sometimes they can be lazy and lack motivation, but they have to have a lot of verbal contact. And with Johnny Carson, he was famous for being a talk-show host. If you are a Libra and you are in an environment with workers who are always arguing, or you're in an ugly, disgusting environment, you could get sick. Or you will become stressed. Libra likes to have nice things around them. I think Leo does also. Any Venus ruled sign has to be in a harmonious environment with pleasant co-workers. The more inharmonious the sur roundings the more acidic you can become over the long term and remember this acidity affects your joints, tissues and bones over time.

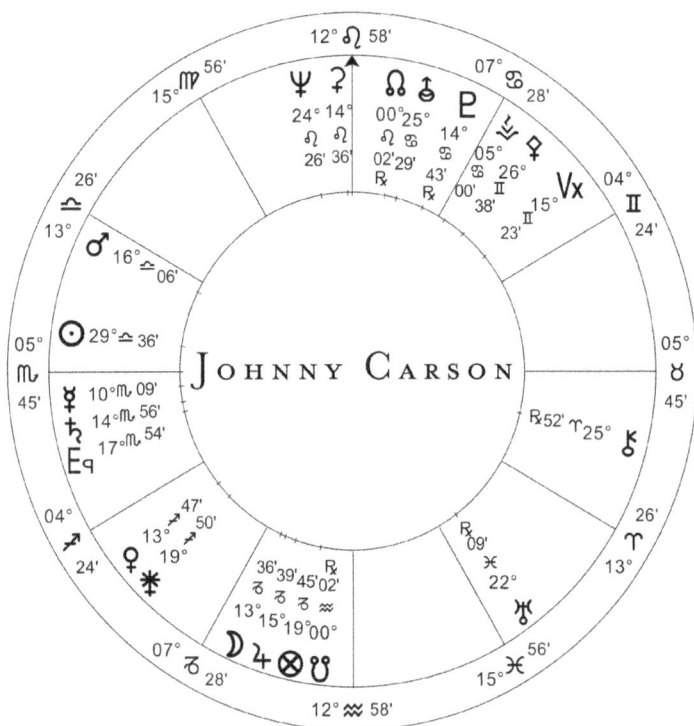

JOHNNY CARSON

The fact that Libras can be very indecisive can cause stress. They also have to learn how to say no. Now, as for Johnny Carson, maybe his shyness was the 29° Sun in the 12th house. There's the glamour and charisma with Neptune at the top of the chart. And the potential for scandal and negative publicity that occurred during one of his divorces. And look at Venus trining the MC from the 2nd house. It's almost exact. This is another indication of wealth. A good aspect between 2 and 10 can bring wealth and prosperity. So he was shy and no one knows a lot about him. Notice the Scorpio rising. He didn't reveal a lot about himself. He was very powerful. So he certainly exhibited being in a Libra profession. However, the profession is not necessarily the Sun sign. I have chosen one of each sign as an illustration but the profession is going to be much more than that. I still think that you need to honor your Sun sign. I heard years ago that it's your path in life, and you must follow it to some extent. I don't care what people say about the Ascendant being more important. If you don't do something involving your Sun, you're not fulfilling your destiny.

SCORPIO

Now we've got Scorpio and the example is Bill Gates. Scorpio needs an intense focus in whatever they do. Something that is high impact. They can take things and themselves too seriously. They can get into power struggles with co-workers. They're another sign that can upset their co-workers, being too blunt or too authoritarian. They're great in a crisis. You can depend on them. And they also like some risk. Scorpio can have extreme mood changes,

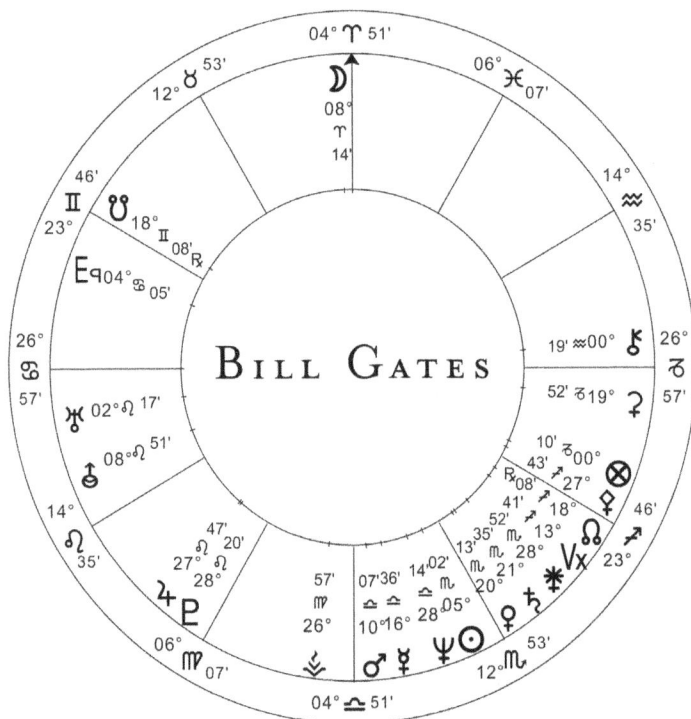

but they need to have time to passionately express themselves in some way. They have to have something they can throw themselves into heart and soul. As for Bill Gates, I heard that he had a bad temper and was moody. That's interesting. Cancer rising. And Sun in Scorpio. That's a good example. The Moon in Aries would add to being emotionally volatile and impatient. I would say that he would be very acidic. The Moon in Aries, the Sun in Scorpio and the Cancer rising for mood changes. There's Uranus in the same sign as his second house cusp. We know how he earned money with Uranus ruling computers and technology. The point is he took everything he had and made it high impact.

SAGITTARIUS

The Sagittarius example is Walt Disney. Sagittarius doesn't always have great staying power. And they need something that allows them to be mobile. I always think of Sagittarius as the rancher. A perfect example of a Sagittarius who would be happy is a rancher as Sagittarius also rules horses. And they like the great outdoors.

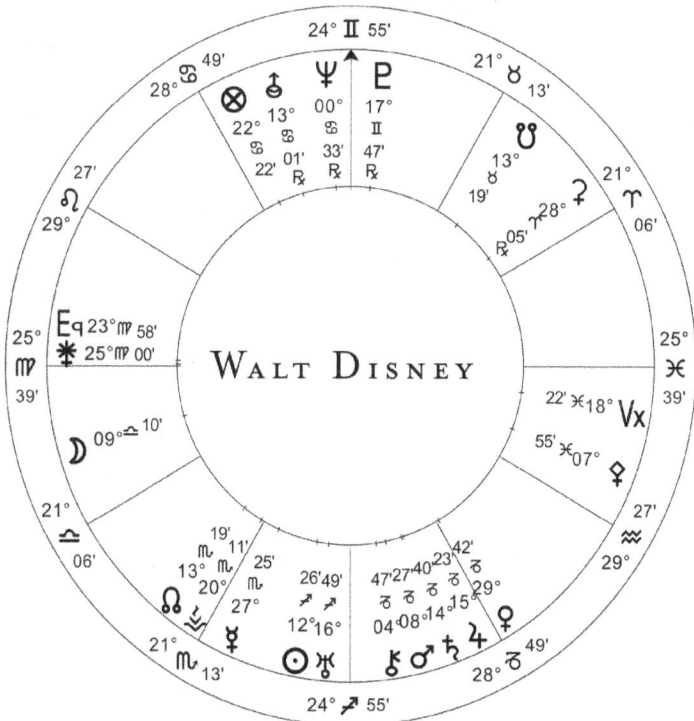

WALT DISNEY

A traveling sales person possibly though that could also be Gemini. Sagittarius doesn't like to be confined to one thing. They get easily bored with everyday environments. They have to have goals. Sagittarius can be an inspirational sign. They have to have diversity and physical exercise. Walt Disney's chart is fascinating. What was he known for? What's at the top of his chart? He was known for fantasy and Neptune is at the top of the chart. And in 00 Cancer no less. Anything in 00 degrees can be something new and fresh. In the early stages. And 00 Cancer is on the world axis so what he did influenced the whole world and connected him with the world at large. He has a Sun Uranus conjunction. I see him as a unique person with vision – the unique vision of Sun conjunct Uranus in Sagittarius with all the glamour of Neptune. And let's not forget Disneyland for a fantasy land. Neptune can be scandal also. And a good example is Jackie Kennedy Onassis with Neptune at the top of her chart. In her case Neptune was a combination of glamour and scandal. And it could also indicate lymphoma which is what she died of. Walt Disney died after suffering cardiac arrest caused by lung cancer.

Audience: He got frozen.

DC: That's right. We should see if anything like that shows in the chart. A Mars Saturn conjunction? However, his family denies this story of him being frozen. Anyway, his is the perfect example of the vision of a Sagittarian.

CAPRICORN

Then we have Capricorn and the example is Joe Frazier, the boxer. Now Capricorn is a perfectionist. And they can be controlling and they dislike change. The more controlling you are, which can be Scorpionic also, the more stress you are placing on your body. So Capricorn can be inflexible, rigid and insensitive at times. I also read somewhere that Capricorn can't stand loud noise. So you don't want to be in an environment that is noisy. They're very good with the use of time. They are self sufficient, and they do need to do exercises that calms, strengthens and refreshes them.

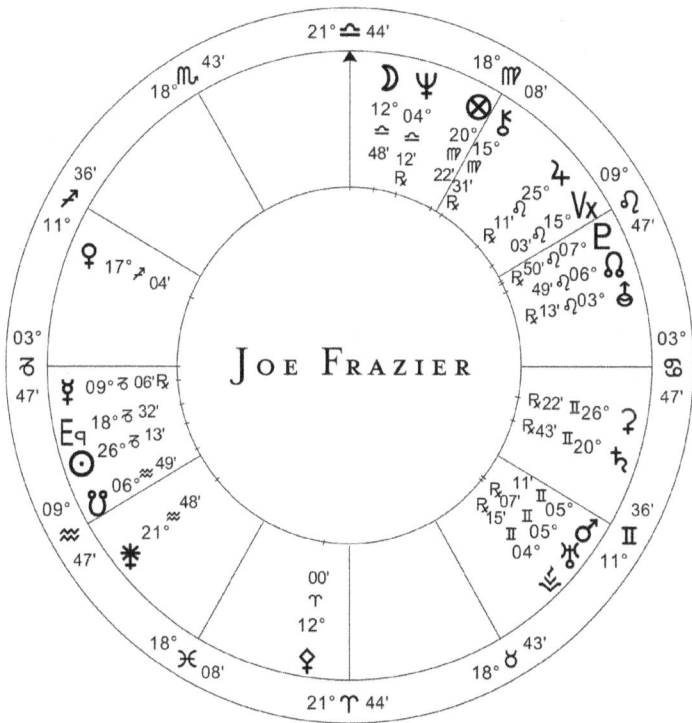

JOE FRAZIER

So Joe Frazier, I don't know if by looking at the chart you see a boxer, but you certainly see control. Anyone who succeeds in boxing has to have some kind of power or strength or endurance, which would be Capricorn. And he has Saturn in the 6th, which also gives you control and endurance in work. Saturn also trines the MC which shows the use of discipline in the career as well as gaining respect. Mars Uranus in Gemini would give him the agility you need in boxing. The Capricorn Sun also indicates he went up the ladder in his profession which is also Capricorn's favorite thing. Getting to the top. And the control.

AQUARIUS

Now Oprah Winfrey is an Aquarian. Aquarius can be very erratic; they can be dreamers. They do what they want to do no matter what people tell them as they are not afraid to be different. And therefore Aquarius has to do something different. They cannot follow the norm. So Oprah Winfrey certainly became unique and look at Jupiter in the 6th for success along with Mercury in the second trine the MC. That would certainly give success as a communicator. And Neptune is at the top for glamour and her involvement with films. She also appeals to the masses, which is very Aquarian. Remember FDR was an Aquarian and he started Social Security. So there's that element of helping the masses. There's more to her than this as there is more to everyone than their Sun sign.

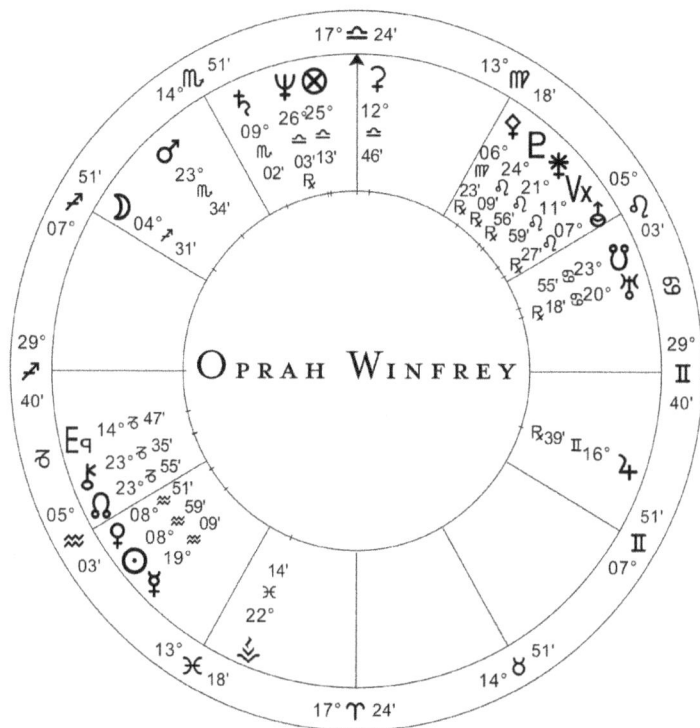

OPRAH WINFREY

PISCES

Pisces has a tendency to space out or get into drugs, alcohol or tobacco, which can definitely contribute to stress. Pisces likes eccentric or off-beat careers. They don't like to be in an occupation that requires toughness; they don't like to be around a lot of noise or chaos. They like their leisure time. And they may not like plain old 9 to 5 jobs. They want to do something with their imagination. And Michael Caine is certainly a good example of Pisces. He has a Sun

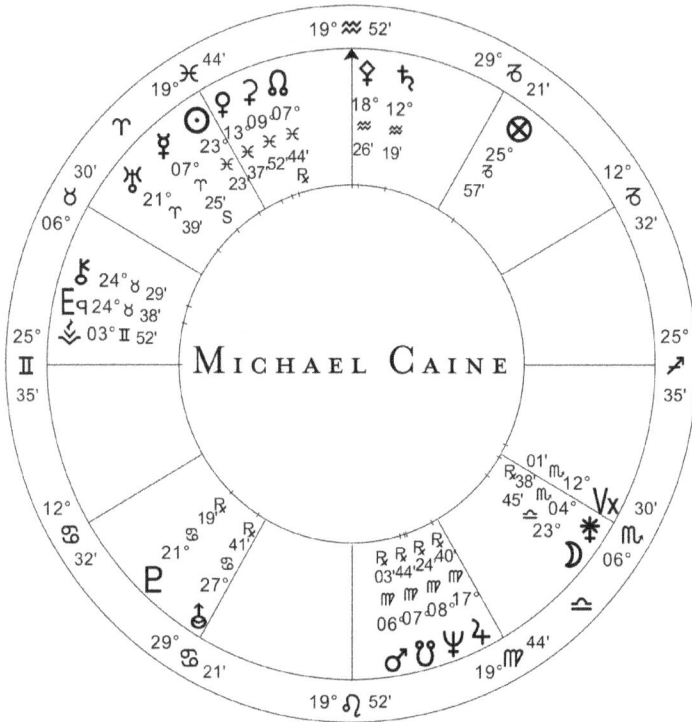

MICHAEL CAINE

in Pisces so he became a film star. That's one good way to use Pisces. Probably the Venus Node in the 10th makes him very likable. That's another helpful combination for earning money. And he has the Moon, ruler of the 2nd house, trine the MC, which is another signature for making money. I think sometimes when you are looking at the chart of a movie star you are seeing the roles they play. He played some pretty tough characters and he has a close Sun trine Pluto aspect. I don't know if anything stands out to you. The Aquarius MC can be a unique profession. With the Pisces Sun one of the things you could choose is film, but it could be many other professions. I think the Moon in Libra is another reason people like him. He's a very likable person and he has had a very long career. Age has not kept him from working and getting parts in movies. That could be Saturn elevated at the top of the chart for security and hard work. The Pisces could indicate his ability to merge into so many roles.

TRANSITS TO CAREER HOUSES

Now let's discuss the type of stress you can experience when the outer planets transit your career houses. There was a book published by Llewellyn in 1992 entitled *How To Use Vocational Astrology for Success in the Workplace*[3] edited by Noel Tyl. And one of the contributing writers, Jayi Jacobs, has a chapter "Career Cycles, Job changes, and Rewards" describing how the planets affect you in the workplace. There is useful information on the transits of the outer planets to 2, 6 or 10, the houses associated with income, work and career. Jacobs includes all the aspects and all the houses if you want more information. I'm just including the vocational houses.

There are certain planets that will cause you more stress than others. I don't think Venus will cause you a lot of stress unless it's from overeating. Pluto certainly can and does. Also Saturn, Uranus and Mars. Pluto can spend from 12 to 14 years in a house and as it transits, you may not notice it as much; you have to live with it. What does Pluto have to do in terms of workplace stress? Obsession. It gets you obsessed; you're getting too stressed. It transforms you. It's a catalyst for change. It compels you to do something. And it can cause a crisis also. It can be a breakthrough too. Pluto can empower you. What happens when it goes through your second house? It can completely change your value system. Jacobs says it can destroy it piece by piece. Nothing has the same worth as before. Pluto going through your second house could cause financial fluctuation. So by the end of the transit you will look back and notice changes in your financial life since Pluto's initial transit.

Pluto transiting the 6th could make your work habits change profoundly. Sometimes Pluto in the 6th could be a health crisis that cripples your career. So obviously that's pretty stressful. Or you crave some type of employment that will fulfill your very existence. I've mentioned that the sixth house, which is supposedly the house of health, has to do with how your day-to-day life or even your working environment causes stress that could lead to illness. Issues involving the sixth house are one of the factors, but not the only factor that leads to a health problem. It is an underlying cause that you need to look at but the sixth house covers day-to-day routines, and if your day-to-day life is stressful, you're building up acid.

Pluto in the 10th could mean you become more ambitious or you change careers. Maybe you will get into a whole new career. Or the career can swallow up your life. And maybe now you're ready to take a risk. It gives a strong drive for success or authority.

Neptune remains around 14 years in a house. It all depends on how fast it is moving and on the size of your natal houses, depending on what house system you use. If you have a large house, obviously the planet will remain in the house longer. When Neptune transits your second house, you may start earning income by giving service to people, or you become more inspired by what you do. Or it could just be economic uncertainly. When people start to become mediums or mystics or psychics, they might have Neptune going into their second house. They also might find an uncertainty with income. It can be something high or something low with Neptune. You really can't tell. The positive part is helping professions. The negative part is uncertainty about income that can lead to stress.

When Neptune goes into the sixth house, you might become more creative at work or possibly something deceptive or underhanded goes on in the workplace. I also find that when Neptune goes into the sixth house, it can indicate allergies. Now sometimes it can describe allergic reactions if you're in a toxic building, because it's the sixth house of work and health and suddenly you develop allergies. Or you suddenly become allergic to a food you normally eat. A fourth house Neptune could also relate to food allergies because the 4th and 10th houses have to do with food intake and assimilation. This is all very general and you have to look at the individual chart. Watch out for food or environmental allergies when Neptune goes into the 6th.

Now when Neptune goes into the 10th house, you might finally find the career you've always wanted – your real calling in life. Or what's the opposite. You don't have the faintest idea of what to do. You're completely confused. Certainly if someone was in the film industry and Neptune went into their 10th house, it could help their career. Somebody who doesn't know where they're going, the situation could get worse.

Now when Uranus transits the work houses it can disrupt or alter. You can reinvent yourself. There can be a new-found independence. Or you rebel against everyday work, and you could quit a job. It will be something unusual, inventive, disruptive, different or independent. If it goes into your second house, there could be shocking changes in your financial situation. Suddenly, you have to reassess your finances. But, positively, it could be a sudden windfall. And you can use all those keywords for Uranus such as working in technology or with computers.

As it goes into the sixth, you could become self-employed. I think there's always erratic hours connected with Uranus, and it also indicates an ability to freelance with the 6th house. You could find that when Uranus goes into your 6th house you cannot stand your day-to-day routines anymore. You've had it with 9 to 5. You change your routines and do something different. So that would be one meaning of Uranus in the 6th, getting into some unusual work that you hadn't expected to do.

In the 10th, something bizarre could happen. Your career could go up; your career could go down. You could get into a new career. You could do something free lance with Uranus in the 10th also. I think the positive thing about Uranus is if you want to work for yourself, it can help as it transits 2, 6 or 10. Either way, you've going to want change and need a new routine. You never know what to expect when it enters the 10th. Jacobs said that you could have real flip-flops, and you could just barely make it by the skin of your teeth with Uranus in the 10th. I'm sure all of you have had some of these transits going through these houses that you can relate to.

And then the other planet I would look at is Saturn. And what do we know about Saturn? It's going to limit, restrict or hold us back in some way or cause us to work harder. And in the second house you may have cash-flow problems or you restructure your values but I don't necessarily think you will have less money. You might be able to start saving. Jacqueline Kennedy Onassis had Saturn in the second house. Never assume that with Saturn in the second you will not have any money. We're trying to look at these planets in terms of causing workplace stress. So Saturn in the second at its worst is a cash-flow problem or not getting what you deserve. Or maybe you're making a lot of money, but it's affecting your health as you're working such long hours. That could be very Saturnian also.

With Saturn transiting the sixth house, you could become ill from stress or working long hours. If the sixth house describes working conditions, then work could become very stressful – burnout, working two jobs, being underpaid, being unappreciated. The sixth house is the kind of daily activity a person should pursue in the course of their work for fulfillment. So if you look at it in a positive way, with Saturn in the sixth you could get more structured at work if you're normally completely disorganized and can't find anything on your desk.

Saturn in the 10th – I always heard it could be a fall from power or you can reach a peak in your career. It could indicate total career absorption. Saturn is also authority, the display of status and being seen as very knowledgeable about your career so people will look up to you.

Those are the planets that I would look at transiting the vocational houses in relation to causing stress. I think Uranus causes the most stress. Those with a strong natal Uranus can't handle stress for long periods of time. Or they overreact when stressed. Or you are very nervous and high-strung all the time. You can't relax. And if you have a strong Uranus in your chart, you need to unwind through exercise, meditation or biofeedback. You could become spastic or develop tics with a strong Uranus. I think Mercury could have a similar effect if strong or afflicted in the chart. And if you have a strong Mercury and Uranus combination, you are in danger of totally stressing yourself out through nervousness and you need to find ways to calm yourself and release tension.

Inner planetary transits can also cause stress. I found some useful information on daily stress in an article in the "Mountain Astrologer"[4]. We just talked about Saturn, Uranus, Neptune and Pluto, which lead to big changes that can take longer to manifest and might not be noticeable right away. If you're looking at transits of the Sun through Mars, you're seeing day-to-day stress. This daily stress can build up and sometimes be as difficult as stress caused by the outer planets.

So the Sun and Mars can be physical stress where you're fighting off a cold or you are physically exhausted or you are pushing yourself too hard. And also Mars transits, and I was thinking of Mercury Mars combinations – you're stuck in traffic and you become really high strung. A daily grind of being stuck in traffic causes stress and causes you to be more acidic. It goes back to the whole acid/alkaline imbalance. You have a Mercury Mars combination by transit in your chart one day, and you go to work and get into an argument with a co-worker, or you do something impulsive that causes a problem. So you can look at your daily transits to see how you are handling day-to-day stress and know that if you drive to work, you are building up stress just by being in traffic. Maybe you could listen to soothing music.

Mars itself can cause ego conflicts, rash behavior, impulsiveness. It gives you the energy you need to get through the day, but it can lead to adrenal insufficiency by pushing yourself too hard.

Solar transits affect your vitality and you don't usually think too much of them. Watch the day that the transiting Sun is on your Saturn and see how you feel – a hard aspect to Saturn from the Sun can indicate less vitality; a hard aspect from the Sun to Neptune could be a minor infection. But, generally speaking, the most stress involving the Sun would be problems with authority figures or conflicts involving the use of the will.

Lunar transits, if you're that anal retentive and you sit there watching your lunar transits every day, can tell you when you might be angry, when you are more relaxed, when you might overeat, etc. I don't know that many astrologers who study their daily lunar transits unless they're looking for a good time to start a project or watching the void Moon. Lunar transits do affect your emotions.

Mercury transits affect your everyday life. What about an upsetting phone call? I have seen some stressful days when Mercury transits in hard aspect to Saturn. Really bad days – how can this supposedly one-day transit of Mercury to my Saturn cause so much trouble? Because something happens and you are stuck with Saturn. And you have to do this and you have to do that. So even a one-day transit of Mercury can cause severe stress. And we're not going to walk around all day being Buddha's and meditating, but you know that saying that you can't change what happens to you, you can only change your reaction to it. That's the message to all of us. Lots of luck.

Venus transits can indicate indulgence or laziness. You don't feel like going to work or sometimes it's a day that you have a financial fluctuation that stresses you out. Or overindulgence in food that leads to indigestion. I didn't mention Jupiter transits, but they can also be periods of overindulgence, overspending or exaggeration.

TREATMENT

I'll give you some treatment ideas based on the planets.

If you have a solar problem, build up your vitality. Do breathing exercises. Or get more sunlight. A little bit of sunlight can help you. Therefore light therapy might also be helpful. Remember what Stephen Arroyo said in *Astrology, Psychology, and the Four Elements* – use the element of your Sun to build up your vitality. This was discussed in Chapter Five: Rebalancing with the Elements and Modes.

Lunar problems respond to water treatment such as hydrotherapy or just good nutrition. Also ingesting more fluids.

Now this is more general medical astrology information than dealing with the topic of workplace stress, but if you have a planet in high focus, you can use that planet to determine how you might be treated. For example, if I see someone with a strong Sun in the chart, I'll use information on treatment involving the Sun. A strong Sun needs to see an expert and needs to build up the vitality. A strong Sun might also respond to Vitamins A and D. Also see a nutritionist as you will be given information unique to you.

Mercury needs to learn about the problem. If you have a disease, get more information about it. Otherwise, do disciplines like yoga and mental and physical exercises that stimulate your mind. With a strong Mercury you will want to be busy and use your mind. And if you think of these planets in terms of work, with a strong Mercury if you're not using your mind or you are stuck at a sedentary job all day, it could lead to illness due to stress. Doing work you hate can lead to illness as hatred increases acid in the body which leads to illness.

Now Venus has to do with diet and nutrition. So if you have a strong Venus in your chart, you need to use therapies that are soothing such as aromatherapy or engage in activities that are pleasurable. Flower essences may help you; also being on a healthy diet.

If you have a very strong Mars and you are very stressed out, you might find that acupuncture helps you as it uses needles and Mars rules needles; also increasing foods containing iron. Eating more meat is a Mars treatment. Martial arts are a good way to use Martian energy; anything aerobic is also good. Lunar treatments can tone down the heat of Mars.

Avoid unhealthy fats and too much fried food if you have a strong Jupiter as you have to be sure to get healthy fats into your diet. And you want to watch your diet. Jupiter will want to do something traditional. A person with an emphasized Jupiter in the chart is not going to look for some weird cure if they have a problem. Jupiter is very conventional. And one cure seems to be a liver tune up if you have a strong Jupiter or an emphasis in Sagittarius in your chart. A liver tune up can help a lot and that type of information is in a lot of health books. I would do it under the supervision of a nutritionist.

Audience: What is a liver tune up?

DC: It is a method of cleansing toxins from the liver. It can involve an avoidance of certain foods and/or an ingestion of certain foods to build up the liver function in the body. It could take a week or two. You can get more information from the books I mentioned or on the Internet. What I never realized before reading the books I mentioned is that there are alkalizing lifestyles.

Saturn has a lot to do with time. If you can control your time, you can remain healthier. Saturn uses items like cold packs, astringents and minerals. And abstinence. And clay. Think of what the planet rules and what it can do for you. The Moon is water and Saturn is the earth so clay and minerals are a Saturn treatment and liquid is a lunar treatment. I also remember reading about mud packs with Saturn. That could be Moon Saturn also.

Anything radical or unusual is Uranus. Anything different. I don't know too much about radionics but it is a controversial Uranian treatment. Also acupuncture. And energy healing.

With Neptune you might need more sleep, meditation. Also aromatherapy and homeopathy. I'm very much into homeopathy. Prayer. All of these are Neptunian. Water therapies are also good for Neptune.

And with Pluto, if you believe in it, past life regression is a cure for Pluto or therapy, especially Gestalt therapy. Psychotherapy. Purification diets, which should be done under supervision. And gender reassignment is Pluto. If you think it will help, you can change your sex.

1   Vasey, Christopher, N.D., *The Acid-Alkaline Diet for Optimum Health.* Healing Arts Press, Rochester, Vermont. English translation 2003.

2   Baroody, Dr, Theodore A., *Alkalize or Die,* Holographic Health Press, Waynesville, NC, 1991.

3   Tyl, Noel (Edited by), *How to Use Vocational Astrology for Success in the Workplace,* Llewellyn Publications, St. Paul, MN, 1992.

4   Kim, Falconer, "Rapid Transits," *The Mountain Astrologer.* Issue 111, October 2003, pg. 82 – 93.

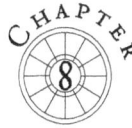

NUTRITIONAL NEEDS
IN THE NATAL CHART

This chapter helps you to identify such complaints as skin problems, constipation, female problems, digestive disorders, gum complaints and hardening of the arteries in relation to nutritional deficiencies and planetary significators. Information on Mars and Saturn in the signs in terms of nutrition is given. There is also a valuable bibliography at the end of this chapter listing astrology books that contain information on nutrition and astrology.

Nutrition is a part of medical astrology but before you even study nutrition in relation to astrology, you've got to use common sense about food and diet. Many people have poor diets. They eat what they like whether or not the food is good for them. I will give you indications in the chart that describe eating habits as well as how to use the signs and planets to determine nutritional deficiencies in the chart.

Now with medical astrology in most cases we're not doctors. You're learning how to see medical issues in a chart but you're not a doctor so you can't diagnose. The same goes for talking to a client about nutrition. If you don't know anything about vitamins and minerals or how food is utilized in the body, you shouldn't be advising clients as if you were a nutritionist. So if you're new at medical astrology, use this information for yourself. I wouldn't use it to advise other people unless you've studied nutrition. I started studying astrology and nutrition at the same time. They both went together for me. And so I have all those years that I've read books on nutrition. I don't think I understood nutrition at the beginning. It's like those first 10 astrology books you started with. You don't understand the first 10 on vitamins and minerals and nutrition either.

So I would say go to the bookstores. In terms of illness some of the problems people have can be attributed to poor nutrition. Nutrition isn't everything. You can't ignore hereditary and lifestyle. And, of course, when you look at the chart, you can see health issues. When people come to see me for a health reading I tell them their strengths and weaknesses and what they're prone to. I can see potential nutritional deficiencies that might help solve some of their problems. I don't know that you can cure diseases just by nutrition, but I think good nutrition helps to keep your body toned and your immunity up.

So you have to read books and magazines and keep up with the latest information on health and nutrition. The first thing you want to know is how to recognize a deficiency or a problem in the chart.

SKIN PROBLEMS

Let's start with skin problems. What can you tell from the chart and what can you do to remedy the situation?

Venus Saturn in hard aspect can indicate skin disorders. Also Saturn in Libra. Or Venus in Libra afflicted. Just because you have Venus in Libra doesn't mean you will have skin problems, but if Venus is afflicted by Mars, you could have skin eruptions. With Pluto even more so as Pluto is a higher octave of Mars. Venus Pluto is also associated with skin growths. Another significator is Saturn in Capricorn as Saturn rules the skin and Saturn problems can sometimes result in dry skin. Also Mars in Aries. That could describe pimples on the face. So let's say you're looking at a chart and you see some of these planetary combinations. You could use essential fatty acids, zinc and Vitamin A.

Use high quality oil too. I hear people saying I'd better not have oil; I'm going to get fat. You need at least a tablespoon a day of oil such as olive oil. You could get skin problems such as dryness or scaling from not ingesting enough oil. PABA, which is one of the B vitamins, is helpful and can also be used as an ointment. And by the way, just because you have the significators doesn't mean you're going to get the problem. If you have the problem, you will usually have some of these significators. With astrology even the most difficult indications in the chart may not manifest into anything serious. Don't forget heredity, your environment and lifestyle.

So you could have Saturn in Libra, Venus in Libra. Again, think of Libra and Capricorn as skin indicators. Also Saturn in Capricorn and Mars in Aries. And they will manifest differently. Skin problems are just a general term. It can be dry skin, psoriasis. It can be eruptions, hives. That's one thing about medical astrology. First you take it generally and then you can get more specific. You fine-tune your work. The addition of Neptune with these significators could indicate that the problem is caused by an allergy or an infection.

Audience: Could this manifest as moles? I know someone with both Saturn and Venus in Libra.

DC: Yes, I think it could. I have cases of moles with Venus Saturn aspects.

Audience: What would it mean if someone told you they have a lot of scratchy places on their back and they were always scratching them? Their skin is erupting on the back.

DC: You mean itching? I still say eruptions are usually Mars in Aries or a Mars Pluto aspect. I don't think it's that simple because if it's caused by some health disorder and the toxins are being eliminated in the skin, you need to find the cause. You look at the rulership of the skin, which is Saturn and see how afflicted it is. It's not that cut and dry. It's never that simple. And again, you need to look at the whole chart. Sometimes you just need to change your laundry detergent.

Audience: Is it your natal chart or where you are now?

DC: It's based on your natal chart. You could have a transit or a progression that involves these same planets and the problem arises now.

CONSTIPATION

Now, a big issue with many people is constipation. So let's see how that shows up in the chart and what you can do about it. You may need more fiber in your diet. You might benefit from more oil and from flaxseed or psyllium. Psyllium is one of the plants used now to balance the body, as it's pretty natural.

How would you recognize this in a chart? Saturn in Scorpio or Saturn in Taurus. Saturn in Virgo is another indicator. Now sometimes constipation is caused by stress – an angular Uranus or Mercury Uranus aspect in hard aspect. Or a lot of mutability in the chart. You have to ask what's causing the problem. Is it caused by stress or is it caused by a problem in the diet? Well, the planets may point out to you the cause. Somebody may say they have this problem and you look at the chart and they have a lot of mutability or an angular Uranus or a Mercury Uranus aspect. You're totally stressed out. Maybe they don't even take enough time for bathroom breaks as they are always in a hurry. Or you might look at the chart and see you have Saturn in Taurus or Saturn in Scorpio or a lot of fixed planets, and the constipation is not caused by stress. There's a problem in elimination and therefore you need foods to bring your body back into balance. You may need more fiber in your diet. Increase fruits and vegetables. Drink more water.

So you have to look at the cause of the problem. And the chart can help you. That's why I'm starting with some basics to give you an understanding. Taurus and Scorpio problems can be significators of constipation.

Audience: What about Saturn in Virgo and Pisces?

DC: Saturn in Virgo and in Pisces tends to be more intestinal although they still all can end up causing constipation. I've categorized it so when it's Saturn in Virgo you may need more enzymes whereas if it's Saturn in Scorpio you may need more fiber. Do you see the difference? In my own mind I try to do it that way because there are differences between the signs. Do you need more fiber? Do you need more enzymes? Do you need both? Is there an enzyme problem? – Saturn in Virgo.

As I've mentioned throughout the book, one rule of thumb in medical astrology is to use the crosses. Is it a cardinal problem, a fixed problem or a mutable problem? The intestines and pancreas are ruled by Virgo which belongs to the mutable cross and Saturn, being the weakest point in the body, you may need enzymes even if you have Saturn in Sagittarius because Sagittarius is also a part of the mutable cross. It sometimes works that way. Though it usually works with the polarities. Most of the time it's the Taurus Scorpio axis or the Virgo Pisces axis for constipation.

FEMALE PROBLEMS

Female problems could be helped by B-complex, vitamin E, potassium, choline and inositol, which is lecithin and calcium and magnesium. By the way there are many books on female problems. I'm just giving you hints. So how would you recognize this in a chart? A Venus Pluto affliction could show up. Every once in a while you see Venus Pluto in a trine and you wonder why the person is experiencing a problem. It's usually a square or a conjunction involving a malefic.

Venus in Scorpio. Moon in Scorpio also. A Moon Venus square or opposition. I don't know about a conjunction. I believe it's more squares or oppositions. Also Saturn in Scorpio. And a combination of Venus, Mars and Pluto can also indicate female problems. I've seen them as a signature for a hysterectomy.

So, again, you look at the planets, which might be describing the problem and you look at what you can do nutritionally. And when I use the words vitamins and minerals, I'm not necessarily saying you should go out and buy vitamins and minerals. I always think you should try to get nutrients from food and use the vitamins and minerals as a supplement. And I take the least amount myself. I never take the most. I've been taking vitamins and minerals for many years, but I've never taken a lot of them. I just take a little every day. And also I try to eat right. And get a good night's sleep. The whole bit. It works.

NUTRITIONAL DEFICIENCIES

Now someone might be complaining of a dry mouth and doesn't realize they're having digestive problems because they are experiencing a lack of hydrochloric acid in the stomach. Saturn in Cancer can indicate poor digestion and sometimes it's Saturn in Capricorn. One of the symptoms is a dry mouth.

Audience: What are they lacking – hydrochloric acid?

DC: Hydrochloric acid, which you can take in tablet form. It's called betaine hydrochloric acid. That is a digestive aid, but if you have a chart that shows a lot of acidity like Mars in Aries or Moon square Mars, you need to be careful of adding more acid into your body. That's why I said the first thing you have to do with nutrition is to use common sense combined with what you see in a chart.

Now liver or gallbladder problems can be helped by Vitamin D which helps produce the bile in the gallbladder. This problem can be shown by Saturn in Sagittarius, a Sun Saturn combination, a Jupiter Saturn combination or Saturn in Capricorn.

Audience: Even trines or sextile?

DC: It's like I said. Most of the time it will be hard aspects but not all the time. Occasionally, you'll see a trine thrown in. You're not going to see a chart that is well aspected getting really difficult problems. If a trine is involved, it's because there's another reason. It's part of a larger configuration in the chart.

I have seen Jupiter Saturn combinations show up with arteriosclerosis, hardening of the arteries or loss of tissue elasticity. Because Jupiter rules the arteries and Saturn is the hardening. So another thing to think about, if you see Saturn and Jupiter in hard aspect in your chart, watch your diet as far as fats as you may be prone to arteriosclerosis or high cholesterol. It seems strange to say this from one aspect but if you've also got problems with Leo and the 5th and 11th houses, add it up – it's a signature for heart disease. One indication does not make a problem just like one transit should not be devastating in your life. You usually need a lot of planetary activity for major events to happen in life.

Audience: Could Saturn in Capricorn be an arthritic problem?

DC: Yes, it could, but usually it would be accompanied by a hard aspect from Mars if it's going to be really serious. It's usually not just one placement. I'm just giving you clues. If you are new to medical astrology and nutrition, these are clues to help you get started. You would be overwhelmed if I went into every little detail. This information along with utilizing the book list at the end of this chapter will give you a greater understanding of astrology and nutrition.

So you read books; you keep up with the latest research. You look at a chart and you see deficiencies. You also have to know about deficiencies that have nothing to do with the chart. People who are on medication can require more vitamins and minerals. Those who live in a poor environment can be nutritionally deficient. Now environmental sensitivities can sometimes show up as Saturn in Aquarius or Saturn Pluto or Saturn Neptune combinations. There's something wrong. You're sensitive to toxins in the air. You're more affected by pollution with these aspects especially those with Saturn in Aquarius. If you smoke, you need more nutrients, more Vitamins A and C, foods such as carrots and broccoli.

Audience: What if you don't smoke and you're asthmatic?

DC: There are nutritional remedies for asthma such as vitamin E, potassium. Possibly acupuncture. And allergies are difficult as it's hard to find the cause. They're not necessarily caused by food.

If you take the birth control pill, you need more B6. If you don't get enough sunshine, you need more Vitamin D and fish. If you drink a lot of coffee, you need thiamine. If you are a heavy drinker, you need more magnesium and thiamine.

If you have Saturn in Taurus you may experience periodontal problems. There are a lot of things you can do to help your gums and teeth and with Saturn in Taurus, you should do something nutritionally for your gums. Take more Vitamin C, bioflavonoids, and take better care of your gums. See a dentist regularly. Saturn in Taurus can be a sign of gum disease.

MARS AND SATURN IN THE SIGNS

Looking at the sign placements of Mars and Saturn in the chart can give you nutritional information. These sign placements can also give information on proneness to various ailments, but this particular information is geared more to nutrition. The sign placement of Saturn is under active and needs nourishment. It gets the least blood supply of any part of your body. So it could be a weak part of the body where illness develops. And Mars is hyper – it's overactive; that part of the body may be prone to hyperactivity. I'll give some examples. Mars can also indicate a part of the body prone to infection. Perhaps you have Mars in Gemini – you could get a lot of colds.

Saturn in Aries could be dental problems. Also sometimes hearing problems. And with its polarity to Libra, there could be weakened kidney function. You can strengthen your teeth by not eating certain foods – such as a lot of sweets and having regular dental checkups. And taking more calcium, for example.

Audience: Is it Mars in Aries?

DC: No, Saturn in Aries. I didn't find that every planet in a sign led to a nutritional problem, but definitely dental problems can occur with Saturn in Aries. There can also be a tendency to headaches. Saturn in Aries can stand for constriction of the head. Feverfew tea may be helpful for migraines. Mars in Aries can be prone to conditions such as headaches and sunstroke also. Some headaches are caused by food allergies. And too much sun can be detrimental to Mars in Aries. The direct heat of an electric lamp can cause dehydration to Mars in Aries. Drink lots of water.

Saturn in Taurus can be eliminative problems; also gum disease. So there are nutritional aids you can do for these conditions which were mentioned previously.

Audience: Is there a connection with the throat?

DC: Yes, the throat can also be weak with Saturn in Taurus. That's where I have Saturn and when I'm stressed I can get throat problems. Or I lose my voice. Sage tea is excellent for sore throats. Mars in Taurus can be prone to acne due to toxins in the colon or there can be a reaction to foods such as chocolate. Again, good nutrition can help.

Saturn in Gemini may experience nervous problems as they don't have enough calcium and manganese. And magnesium also.

Audience: The lungs also?

DC: Yes, but as far as the lungs go, don't smoke. Both Mars in Gemini and Saturn in Gemini can experience lung problems. Mars in Gemini can indicate lung inflammation and Saturn in Gemini points to the lung area as being weak. Wintergreen tea is useful to nourish the lungs. White onions also aid the lungs.

Mars in Cancer – too much hydrochloric acid. Previously, we said that Saturn in Cancer is not enough hydrochloric acid. If you have Mars in Cancer you're more prone to ulcers. You have to watch what you eat. Be careful of citrus fruits on an empty stomach. Don't push your stomach too much because it's over active. Be careful of too much roughage. This is a case of where you may not want too much roughage where if you had Saturn in Cancer, you may need more stimulation. You have to think of it that way. One is overactive; one is under active. A poor digestive indicator is Saturn in Cancer. You might have poor digestion due to a lack of hydrochloric acid. You need to stimulate your stomach. Cold water before meals stimulates the stomach if you have Saturn in Cancer. Also grapefruit juice. Saturn in Cancer may crave unhealthy food and eat too much cream, sugar or unhealthy desserts.

Mars in Leo can be prone to high blood pressure. Raw garlic can be effective in bringing down high blood pressure. In any case you need to see a doctor if you experience high blood pressure. Mars in Leo is also prone to sunstroke.

Now with Saturn in Leo there is the potential for hardening of the arteries. That's where you should eat a proper diet that is good for the heart. Every chart you look at with Saturn in Leo will not have a heart problem but some will and there are specific diets that are good for you if your chart shows the possibility of heart disease. It's certainly not going to be a problem with every chart. Saturn in Leo can also refer to back problems. Also Saturn in Leo can benefit from calcium and magnesium and potassium for the heart. The heart needs to be stimulated if you have Saturn in Leo. You really need exercise.

Mars in Virgo can indicate an overactive pancreas. Vitamin B, iron, zinc and raw foods are aids to the pancreas.

With Saturn in Virgo, you may go back and forth between diarrhea and constipation. You may need pancreatic enzymes. There can be liver dysfunction. There is a need for intestinal stimulus. You can take pancreatic enzymes just the way you can take hydrochloric acid – in pill form. You also need to eat raw fruits and vegetables if you have Saturn in Virgo to keep your intestines working up to par.

Mars in Libra sometimes leads to kidney inflammation. It can even indicate adrenal exhaustion and skin eruptions caused by kidney dysfunction. Black, red and white currants help treat skin disorders. The adrenals benefit from Vitamin A, Vitamin C, pantothenic acid, zinc and parsley.

Saturn in Libra needs to be careful of hard water building up leading to calcium deposits in the body that affect the kidneys. There can be kidney blockage or gravel or stones of a calcium nature. Corn silk tea and pear juice are useful stimulants for the kidneys.

Mars in Scorpio can be an indication of prostate problems in men. Helpful to the prostate are pumpkin seeds, sunflower seeds, tomatoes, magnesium and zinc. There can also be urinary disorders and female disorders. Red raspberry leaf is an excellent herb for women as well as for urinary tract disorders.

Saturn in Scorpio was mentioned previously. You should consume foods high in fiber for constipation. Mars in Sagittarius is similar to Mars in Gemini in that there can be respiratory disorders. The herbs yarrow and skullcap are useful for respiratory disorders as well as is rosehip tea.

Saturn in Sagittarius like Saturn in Gemini can indicate poor lung capacity. Saturn in Sagittarius can also indicate chronic sciatica problems that can be helped by garlic, iodine or Vitamin B1. I mentioned Saturn in Capricorn – dry skin. It can also be an indication of a sluggish gallbladder. Parsley, wild yams, carrot juice before meals as well as lemon juice are a few remedies for a sluggish gallbladder. Mars in Capricorn can describe eruptive skin disorders and inflammation of the gallbladder. Calendula lotion can be useful to treat skin disorders.

Saturn in Aquarius can lead to anemia or blood problems. Also circulatory problems and oxygenation problems. It's a difficult place for Saturn. One may experience headaches. You need fresh air and foods that are high in iron. There are many types of anemia. You can't just tell a client they have anemia. You have to see a doctor for the specific type of anemia. You can only talk in a general way. If someone is complaining of being tired, you might say you could be anemic. Red Clover tea is considered a blood builder. Rubbing warm coffee grounds on the skin can improve circulation. Mars in Aquarius can also benefit from a blood builder. Wheat grass juice, beets and carrots are also good. Mars in Aquarius is also prone to varicose veins that can be helped by Vitamin E, Vitamin C, calcium and the B vitamins.

Mars in Pisces might experience sugar ailments. There also can be hyperactivity in the intestines and possibly bowel inflammation. Also infectious problems. Foods that help increase healthy bacteria in the intestines include yogurt, kefir and buttermilk. Bananas are excellent for the bowels.

Audience: What about Saturn in Pisces?

Saturn in Pisces is the opposite. You need to be on a diet that builds up your immune system if you have Saturn in Pisces. You can contract colds, flu's, that sort of thing. There can be problems with the white blood cell count. That is one placement where there are lots of books on the market on how to build up your immune system. Astragalus, rosemary, garlic, rose hips, and bioflavonoids are immune enhancers.

DEFICIENCY STATES

The chart can be used to recognize deficiency states. You also need to recognize causative factors that are not in the chart. A person's lifestyle can contribute to a deficiency.

One of the issues with food is how it gets assimilated. Therefore you could be eating all the right foods but have poor assimilation. You may have Saturn in Cancer or Capricorn or in Virgo or Pisces – one of those four placements. You may lack pancreatic enzymes or have low stomach acid. The body needs calcium and iron for acids to digest foods. There may not be enough acid for digestion of proteins and minerals. There is a build up of unhealthy intestinal bacteria in the body so you're getting sick from toxins. You may benefit from apple cider vinegar for an acid deficiency.

Here's some information on minerals taken from http://www.brianmac.co.uk/minerals.htm.

The trace minerals are iron, zinc, copper, selenium, iodine, fluorine and chromium. The major minerals are sodium, potassium, calcium, phosphorus, magnesium, manganese, sulphur, cobalt and chlorine.

Function

- They provide structure in forming bones and teeth
- They help maintain normal heart rhythm, muscle contractility, neural conductivity, and acid-base balance
- They help regulate cellular metabolism by becoming part of enzymes and hormones that modulate cellular activity

Minerals cannot be made in the body and must be obtained in our diet. The daily requirements of minerals required by the body can be obtained from a well balanced diet. Like vitamins, excess minerals can produce toxic effects.

I have a list of minerals from the most to the least absorbable. You see supplements on the market all the time, but you don't know what to buy. The least absorbable are sulfates. We'll go from the least absorbable to the most absorbable. Then chlorides, oxides, carbonates, gluconates, oratates, absorbics with amino acid chelates being the most absorbable. So if you're feel you're not fully absorbing minerals, look at the ones low on the list, chlorides, oxides, carbonates and head toward gluconates, oratates, absorbics and amino acid chelates. There are also a lot of web sites offering minerals with varying claims on their ability to absorb.

Audience: Citrates are also very absorbable.

DC: When you are learning about vitamins and minerals you need to understand their functions in the body. And they all have different functions. My first book *How to Give an Astrological Health Reading (AFA)*, has a section on nutrition. I spent a long time thinking about vitamins and minerals and their relationship to astrology. You open up all these astrology books, and they may have one planet that rules all these vitamins and minerals. I didn't think it made any sense as I felt it was combinations of planets since the vitamins and minerals rule a combination of functions.

In terms of medical astrology, many people experience stress. What can you do for stress? B-complex and magnesium are two supplements considered to be helpful for combating stress. So how would you figure out the rulership. Every planet does not rule B-complex. I divided it up into B1, B2, etc. according to the uses in the body. So you may have an angular Uranus. You may require more B-complex. You may have hard aspects to Mercury. You may have a cardinal emphasis in the chart where you overdo it or a mutable emphasis where you're running on nervous energy. You might have a Mercury Mars or a Mercury Uranus aspect and that's how I went about deciding on what vitamins and minerals you might need. And I can think of more things to add to the list since my first book came out, but if you understand what vitamin helps with a certain function and what planet or combination of planets might indicate the problem, you start to think it through. For example, a person might say they have energy problems; I need vitamin A; my Sun is afflicted. That type of issue. And as I said, in many cases I use combinations of planets to rule various vitamins and minerals the way we use combinations in the chart.

THE HOUSES AND SIGNS IN REGARD TO EATING HABITS

How can you look at a chart and tell your eating habits: There is more than one way and most likely you need to look at a combination of factors such as your Sun, Moon and Ascendant. You can look at the second house for taste and the sixth house for your eating habits and the conditions at mealtime. The second house is the natural house of Taurus which is associated with your taste buds. The sixth house describes your daily routines that includes eating. What kind of eater are you? Look at the cusp of the sixth house. What's an Aries eater like? They may not spend a lot of time at meals. They like hot and spicy food. They may gobble down their food. They may not enjoy cooking or they overcook their food. And they like protein. And Aries may need more food that's high in iron or may require more meat. Some signs do require more meat than other signs.

Taurus is the gourmet who may eat very slowly, and they like to have dessert and that can contribute to weight gain. Gemini eats when they feel like it and they may snack and eat a little bit of this and a little bit of that. They like to talk during mealtime and they need a balanced diet. Cancer enjoys good food and likes to have the family around for dinner. They have traditional tastes and have a lot of pride in what they put on the table. They may have a lot of recipes. And dairy products are an important part of their meal.

This isn't necessarily your Sun sign. This is the sign on your sixth house cusp with an influence from the sign on your second house. You can definitely see a bit of your sun sign in this too. Leo likes food well cooked and hot, warm surroundings, lavish meals and may like to entertain during meals or have a lot of company. Virgo may be the family dietician. They may have a strict dietary regimen, and they like their meals on time or on a very fixed schedule. Libra's like sociability and conversation at mealtime. They may have a sweet tooth and like candy; they may actually enjoy the entertainment part of the meal more than the food itself as it's a chance to socialize. Scorpio doesn't mind eating alone or with one other person. They like to have a drink with a meal, alcohol or otherwise. And they like eating in dark, intimate places. Sagittarius likes a lavish spread. They may have their in-laws as guests; they may overeat and may like foreign or exotic food. Capricorn is very careful of what they eat. They are concerned with form, manners and how the meal is served. They know good food and are excellent coffee and wine tasters. Aquarius may like to experiment with new and unusual dishes, and they may be budget conscious. Pisces eats when they feel like it; they like alcohol and can be fish eaters. And they may enjoy cooking for or entertaining others at meals and may over salt their food.

Audience: Do you also look at the sixth house for potential health problems?

DC: As I've said earlier, I don't use the sixth house that much for potential health problems. It tends to be more functional disorders. Sometimes people look at the sixth house and feel it shows everything, but you have to look at malefics to the angles and know what the signs on the angles rule. When I give my introductory lecture on medical astrology I spend a lot of time explaining afflictions to the angles. I gave some examples in Chapter Six:

"Health Disorders and Addictions and Stressors in the Natal Chart." It's using afflictions to the angles including the vertex to determine proneness to certain types of diseases because the angles are where the problems lie. For example, if you had Leo rising with a square from Saturn in your chart that would indicate a proneness to problems in the fixed cross as Leo is part of the fixed cross.

The sixth house can give you information on your health, but it is not the same as looking at the angles to see what you're prone to. That's been my experience, but I think that every astrologer has his or her own method of looking at a chart as it's partly our intuition we're using. So you have to take that into account.

THE ELEMENTS

You can learn a lot in terms of nutritional needs just by looking at the elements fire, earth, air and water in the chart. You add up points and see if there is an emphasis in a particular element. You're really looking at too much or too little of an element. If you have a reasonable amount of points in a particular element, it is not a problem. You're only looking at an abundance of or not enough of an element. Refer back to Chapter Five: "Rebalancing with the Elements and the Modes" for a complete discussion of the elements.

THE PLANETS

A planet standing out in a chart or a particular planetary combination can give you some kind of nutritional information. How do you know if a planet is strong or weak in a chart? The most elevated planet in a chart is strong. The most angular planet is strong. Your Sun, Moon and the ruler of the Ascendant are strong. If these planets are badly aspected or poorly placed, there can be health problems. The Sun and Moon in angular houses and not afflicted can give strength and energy.

THE SUN

A weak Sun or the Sun being hit by difficult transits or progressions can cause energy problems so you may need something to help your vitality – vitamin A, niacin, thiamine, or phosphorus-containing foods. And sometimes problems with the Sun show a problem with the heart. So you can benefit from more calcium, magnesium, copper, vitamin A and vitamin E. When you are putting this information together, if you also have afflictions to the Sun in Leo, the fifth house, etc. then you can say that the chart shows a potential for heart disease. If it's just one thing with the Sun, it's probably going to be an energy problem. It's doubtful it's a heart problem. Because the Sun seems to show our energy levels more than any other planet, how much energy we have. In difficult combination with the Moon, there can be eye problems. There are supplements on the market to strengthen the eyes. Mars may show more how you use your energy.

There are foods that are ruled by the Sun – rice, sunflowers, grapes and walnuts. So you might try eating more of those foods if you have an afflicted Sun.

THE MOON

The Moon is associated with the water content of the body. An afflicted Moon can indicate a problem with the sodium-potassium balance in the body. The Moon rules mucous formation that is helped by Vitamin A. If the mucous membranes in the body are not kept moist, germs can enter the body, which is why the nostrils should be kept moist. You can use glycerin if you are in a dry room. You just take some glycerin on a Q-tip and put it very lightly around the opening of your nose, and it will keep your nose moist. And if you see problems with the Moon such as a Moon Saturn aspect or the Moon in Capricorn, you may have problems with mucous formation in the body.

The Moon is involved with digestion in the body so problems with the Moon can indicate digestive problems. You may need more potassium and manganese. I touched on digestion at the beginning of this chapter also. Lunar foods are cabbages, the cresses, cucumbers, lettuce, melon and pumpkin. So these foods will help you build up the lunar function.

MERCURY

Mercury, in general, has a lot to do with the nervous system and B-complex vitamins and magnesium. Mercury can indicate problems with mental health when it's afflicted which can also be related to a deficiency of the B-vitamins in the body. Sometimes mental health problems are caused by a nutritional deficiency. It takes a lot of searching and testing to find out the cause. You can be helped by manganese. Your nervous system can be helped in general by calcium, magnesium and B-complex. Mercury has a lot to do with the hormonal system in the body. The endocrine system is not an easy subject for the layperson. There are nutritional remedies given for problems with hormones. Mercury foods are hazelnuts, beans, mushrooms, fennel and pomegranates.

VENUS

Venus rules sugar. As previously mentioned, Jupiter rules fat. They both are involved in weight gain but the weight gain could be caused by sugar if there is a Venus emphasis in the chart or by fat if there is a Jupiter emphasis in the chart.

Again, Venus problems can be sugar problems such as hypoglycemia. You may have a lack of chromium in the body. You need more phosphorous. Venus rules starches also and you may have a problem with how you metabolize starches. And Venus problems can also be helped with Vitamin E. Some foods related to Venus include gooseberry and other berries, wheat, and most of the spices. The real hot spices are associated with Mars.

MARS

Mars is a major player in any chart. Mars is the second planet I would look at for vitality problems. You also judge it along with the Sun to see how you metabolize food. A well-placed Mars fights diseases. A poorly placed Mars has less resistance to disease. If you have a very afflicted Mars, you may need more calming foods. You might be better avoiding a lot of spices. Mars can show blood problems as it rules the red blood corpuscles. Again, that's something only a doctor can tell you. Dandelion root tea is good for purifying the blood. It tastes a bit like coffee and you want the roasted root. It is sometimes used as a coffee substitute.

If you are having a problem with the red blood cells, you may need more B-12 or folic acid. Sometimes Mars can show infection. You need more Vitamin A, Vitamin C, pantothenic acid. Mars rules our muscles. Comfrey leaves can be used as a poultice for sore muscles. Potassium and calcium also help. One of today's most common problems, stress, is related to Mars which rules the adrenals. There is all this talk about adrenal insufficiency caused by stress. Mars in Pisces, a Mars Neptune aspect; an afflicted Mars in Aries or Libra can show problems with the adrenals. Pantothenic acid can aid the adrenals. Mars rules iron metabolism. If afflicted, you may need more copper, molybdenum, and it also has to do with the metabolism of zinc. So it's a very important planet to look at medically speaking. They are all important but Mars gives you a lot of information on how well you are metabolizing, how your fight disease and how you resist disease, along with the Sun. Foods of Mars include chives. Now this would be a weak Mars helped by Mars' foods. Also onions, leeks, peppers, radishes and rhubarb.

JUPITER

Jupiter is involved with fat assimilation. An afflicted Jupiter may need more inositol or manganese. You may have high cholesterol, which could be helped by inositol and choline as well as being on a low fat diet. And you may need more niacin. Again, I said earlier that it seems to be

Jupiter Saturn that shows up with arteriolosclerosis. Foods of Jupiter include chervil, endive, asparagus and figs.

SATURN

Now Saturn, as I said, can give you clues to the weakest part of the body – the sign it's in and the sign opposite. I think that what happens with Saturn is that it is a part of the body that fails first and you may be able to see a cause by looking at Saturn's placement.

Saturn has to do with mineral depletion. And I think that sometimes when you are getting difficult Saturn transits, you need more minerals. It has to do with bruising – you may need more Vitamin P, which are the bioflavonoids. It rules the bones and teeth. You may need more Vitamin C to help assimilate calcium. You may not be absorbing calcium well if you are having bones and teeth problems. Saturn has to do with the hair, skin and nails. And an afflicted Saturn may benefit from iodine, zinc and sulphur.

Saturn foods are barley, beet root and safflower. Also potatoes, parsnips and spinach.

URANUS

I don't have foods for the outer planets but Uranus can have to do with stress, circulation and insomnia. You can benefit from more B-complex. Chamomile tea is good; passion flower is good which you can take as an herbal tea or in capsule form if you feel stressed and have trouble sleeping. And vitamin P and niacin for circulation with Uranus because Uranus rules Aquarius, which rules circulation.

NEPTUNE

Neptune's sign placement is more general, but the sign it occupies can indicate a lack of tone in that part of the body. It is very similar to Saturn since that part of the body can be weak too and needs to be stimulated or nourished. For example, if you have Neptune in Virgo, you may need some kind of intestinal stimulus.

A strong Neptune can describe a person who is drug sensitive. You may need a lower dosage of drugs. You are much more sensitive to drugs including over-the-counter drugs. You can be prone to the bad effects of pollution. A health problem could be caused by toxic metals in your body.

Neptune has to do with the immune system and you need more vitamins A and C when Neptune is afflicted.

PLUTO

Pluto has to do with enzyme action in the body, which can be helped by copper and magnesium. Pluto problems can indicate a need to be detoxified: You can be helped by Vitamin B15, Vitamin E and selenium or just a detoxifying diet. Pluto is a higher octave of Mars. It can be a more massive infection. If Mars is a two-day infection, Pluto is a two-month infection depending. They are similar in that they both rule infection.

Audience: I had a question on what you said about Mars being afflicted and dignified. If it's well aspected are you a better fighter?

DC: Yes, and a resistor.

Audience: When Mars is afflicted is it less resistance?

DC: When Mars is afflicted there can be a lowered immune function. The most difficult are Mars Saturn and Mars Neptune combinations. A well aspected Mars in a fire or air sign is beneficial. It doesn't mean you won't ever get ill; it means you will recover quicker. People who have a strong Mars influence or Aries influence can get a high fever and they may not be that sick. It's just how their body burns off toxins. When Capricorn gets a high fever, it is more serious. When a fire sign gets a high fever, it may not be as serious as an earth sign. Obviously you need immediate medical help if you have a persistent, high fever.

Audience: I've had a long-term problem with dairy products. There's a controversy about them, and I'm especially interested in that I have a child and in giving her milk. What's the connection that you know about between mucous in the body and the use of dairy products?

DC: Astrologically, it can involve a number of factors. Afflictions in the mutable cross could indicate problems with the lungs and a need to keep dairy products low. Allergies to dairy products could show up as afflictions in the cardinal cross or the signs Cancer or Capricorn. Any strong placement of the Moon or Neptune can indicate allergies but not necessarily to dairy products. If you have cardinal planets or the cardinal cross is emphasized, you probably have more trouble with dairy products. Saturn in Cancer could indicate a problem in digesting dairy products. It's not cut and dry. Astrology is a tool but you need a nutritionist and a doctor to get right down to it. The chart can point the way.

You can look at a chart and see how a person should be treated. I described this in Chapter Five: "Rebalancing with the Elements and the Modes." For example, if you have a strong Jupiter, you benefit from using traditional methods. If you have a strong Uranus, you might benefit from acupuncture or very radical methods. If you have Pluto strong in your chart, past life regression or therapy. A strong planet in the chart can point the way to treatment. Saturn would also be very traditional. It could also indicate a need to be more disciplined in diet and exercise. Neptune could be biofeedback and meditation. So you can also look for clues on the best way to treat yourself.

I want to repeat what I said at the beginning of the chapter. Use common sense involving nutrition and food. Listen to your body. You are either in touch with your body or you're not in touch with your body. If you don't have a lot of earth, you're probably not that in touch with your body. If you are aware, you will intuitively know what is good for you and what isn't. What's the best time to eat? How much exercise do I need? And then you can use your chart to say, "I'd better build up this part of my body as I'm weak here. I need this nutrient." You have to keep up with your studies and read a lot to understand nutrition. If every cure worked, we wouldn't have so much sickness. What works for one person, doesn't necessarily work for another. And you also have to consider the planetary influences at a particular time. That's how I look at all this. I try to use common sense combined with astrological knowledge.

REFERENCES FOR CHAPTER 8, AND GENERAL BIBLIOGRAPHY OF MEDICAL ASTROLOGY BOOKS THAT CONTAIN INFORMATION ON ASSESSING NUTRITIONAL NEEDS IN THE HOROSCOPE.

1. Cramer, Diane: *How To Give An Astrological Health Reading,* AFA, Tempe, AZ, 1996.

2. Cramer, Diane: *Managing Your Health and Wellness,* Llewellyn Publications, Woodbury, MN, 2006.

3. Davidson, William: *Davidson's Medical Astrology,* Astrological Bureau, Monroe, New York, 1979.

4. Garrett, Helen Adams, *The Horoscope and the Appetite,* A is A Publishing, Belleville, IL, 1997.

5. Geddes, Sheila: *Astrology and Health,* The Aquarian Press, Wellingborough, Northhamptonshire, 1984.

6. Harmon, J. Merrill: *Complete Astro-Medical Index,* Astro- Analytics Publications, Van Nuys, California, 1979.

7. Jansky, Robert Carl: *Astrology Nutrition & Health,* Para Research, Rockport, Massachusetts, 1977.

8. Jansky, Robert Carl: *Introduction To Holistic Medical Astrology,* American Federation of Astrologers, Inc., Tempe, Arizona, 1983.

9. Jansky, Robert C.: *Modern Medical Astrology,* Astro- Analytics Publications, Van Nuys, California, 1978.

10. Johnson, Kathleen: *Celestial Bodies,* Pocket Books, New York, 1987.

11. Muir, Ada: *Healing Herbs,* Llewellyn Publication, St. Paul, Minnesota, 1995.

12. Nauman, Eileen: *The American Book Of Nutrition & Medical Astrology,* Astro Computing Services, San Diego, CA, 1982.

13. Ridder-Patrick, Jane: *A Handbook Of Medical Astrology,* Arkana, London, England, 1990.

14. Starck, Marcia: *Astrology Key To Holistic Health.* Seek-It Publications, Birmingham, Michigan, 1982.

CHAPTER
9

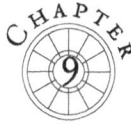

PREDICTIONS AND YOUR HEALTH

NOTE: The following suggestions of herbs and homeopathic remedies are not a substitute for a medical diagnosis or checkup. Always see your doctor if you suspect you have a health problem.

This chapter will combine predictive techniques with the use of homeopathy and cell salts. I recently began studying homeopathy, which matches your symptoms with the remedy. I did this because when my first book was republished *(How To Give An Astrological Health Reading)*, the AFA asked me to write a chapter on homeopathy. When you use homeopathic remedies, you have to take into account the symptoms as well as the major problem along with personality characteristics and time of day the symptoms manifest or are the most pronounced.

Say you're getting a Saturn Neptune combination by transit. That can cause a lot of anxiety. So you look up "anxiety" in a book of homeopathic remedies. And it will list remedies for anxiety. Boiron puts out a free booklet of various symptoms. Sometimes you can find this booklet at a health food store. (See their 800 number under References.) You can also find homeopathic remedies in the health food stores that list symptoms such as anxiety. There are hundreds of remedies that combine various symptoms, but we're just looking at this in a general way. You need a homeopathic practitioner for more help. When you're looking at your own particular symptoms to try to pick a remedy you will find it can be as specific as stating that the symptoms are improved by fresh air and worsened by heat or vice versa. Or it's worse in the morning and better in the afternoon, etc. This is how detailed homeopathy gets.

The difference between homeopathy and allopathy, which is traditional medicine, is that allopathy seeks to suppress the symptoms and homeopathy stimulates the symptoms.

What is homeopathy? Homeopathy was used mostly in the 1800's but it goes back to Hippocrates in that it is a system based on "the law of similars," meaning you use a remedy that has the properties of the symptoms. And how do they know which remedy works? Homeopathic practitioners gave particular remedies to people in good health who produced the symptoms that correspond with the remedy prescribed for those symptoms. Like cures like. And that's how they know what to give a patient.

In other words homeopathy seeks to treat with a similar remedy so as to support the problem. For example, if you have a fever or inflammation then the cure must be a remedy that produces a similar condition in a healthy person. If you have a particular muscle pain, then the remedy should also produce a similar pain in a healthy person. However, even though it produces the condition it should do it without seriously aggravating the condition. The cure should help the person to combat the disease.

Medicine that we use today suppresses the symptoms. If you have a headache, let's get rid of it. Homeopathic remedies stimulate the symptoms and bring them out. It's like an irritant that causes you supposedly to be cured.

So why isn't everybody using homeopathic remedies? Two reasons. The first was the use of antibiotics with the discovery of penicillin. Homeopathy began to go out of style around the time penicillin was discovered. It is still used extensively in Europe and only beginning now to get popular in the United States.

The other reason appears to be the AMA. This is because homeopathic remedies are inexpensive, and you don't need a prescription to use them. So there's no money in them. So those are two reasons I know of why they went out of favor.

Audience: They don't always work. They're not always that effective.

DC: I think they work before you get into deep trouble with a disease. That's what I think about the use of cell salts that we will talk about.

Audience: There might be reasons why they don't work.

DC: Right. You could be taking the wrong remedy. And they are supposed to be non-toxic which is the difference between allopathic medicine and homeopathic remedies. The remedy may not always work, but it's not supposed to have any side effects where regular medicine has known side effects in some people.

And the idea of the law of similars goes way back in time. I'll give you an example. There's a homeopathic remedy called Coffea cruda that is used if you experience insomnia. Normally, you would drink coffee and get insomnia, but the remedy itself stops the insomnia. It is used for people who suffer from nervousness, hypersensitivity and headaches. Let's say you are getting a Uranus transit. You could try Coffea cruda.

The reason I wanted to talk about the cell salts along with homeopathic remedies is that they are easier to use and understand as there are just 12 of them where there are hundreds of homeopathic remedies. And unless you are an expert, you shouldn't be diagnosing yourself.

In 1996 "The Mountain Astrologer" put out an issue with an article on a homeopathic approach to astrology. So you may be able to find this issue on their website – mountainastrologer.com. The article cited a couple of cases. They treated a woman who was having a difficult Saturn transit. And they discussed the Saturnian vibration and recommended two remedies for depression. And they talk about how they treated this woman. So this is a good source to learn about astrology and homeopathy.

Another good source to learn about the cells salts is *The Biochemic Handbook*. This book has been around a long time. It contains many common ailments along with the appropriate cell salt to take along with remedies for different areas of the body that could have a problem. I'll be going thorough the 12 cell salts.

The Biochemic Prescriber is another source of information on cell salts. *The Family Guide to Homeopathy* is useful also. It suggests specific remedies. For example, you could be having a Uranus transit to your Mercury and you can't sleep. What should you do? You look up insomnia and it gives specific times you may be waking up – after midnight, between 1 and 2 am, etc. sleeplessness after 3 am. It gives different homeopathic remedies depending on when your sleeplessness occurs. This is why homeopathy is so involved and so specific. Symptoms also include sleeplessness due to anxiety or sleeplessness due to grief, due to overexcitement, due to overwork, due to racing thoughts. Other symptoms include inability to get back to sleep after waking, talking in your sleep and unusual sleepiness in the morning.

I would read the remedies and see which one fits your symptoms. Homeopathic remedies take into account personality characteristics as well as symptoms. Allopathic medicine doesn't usually take into account personality traits, just what's wrong with you. Suppress it and get rid of it.

Although I am all for regular medicine, I just think there's a way we can incorporate both allopathic medicine and homeopathic remedies in our lives. I think of everything as preventative. Try not to get to the point where you've let your health go. And I think the cell salts help stimulate the body and bring you back to good health.

I think cell salts contain trace elements. There are trace minerals so possibly the cell salts contain trace elements that vitalize the cells in your body and lead to good health. This is also how they are described in the books.

KALI PHOSPHATE – ARIES

Kali Phosphate is the Aries cell salt. It is a brain and nerve builder. It is excellent for your nervous system. What's the planet that could cause nervous problems? Uranus. If you are getting a Uranus transit, this could help you. Even a difficult transit or progression from Mercury can lead to nervousness and anxiety. Kali Phos supplies oxygen in the body. It is useful for mental fatigue that could occur with a transit from Saturn to Mercury. Nervous exhaustion – Uranus Mercury combinations.

Now when I use the planets, I am using them in combinations. It could be a transit, a solar arc, a progression. Just think of these as astrological combinations that produce these symptoms.

Headaches caused by too much study. Mental depression. These can be helped by Kali Phos. It recharges you.

Hysteria. Being fearful or despondent. So it could be helpful during a difficult Saturn transit. It is considered the nerve nutrient. Nervous disorders are usually a combination of Mercury Uranus or Mercury being hit by outer planets. Neptune Mercury could indicate weak nerves. Mercury is the general ruler of the nervous system.

NATRIUM SULPHURICUM – TAURUS

This is the Taurus cell salt. Some practitioners think you should take daily the cell salt ruled by your sun sign and the sign opposite your Sun. Some think you need the cell salt associated with the sign of your South Node or where Saturn is in your chart. I feel you should just take the cell salt associated with a particular symptom or a weakness in the body.

Nat Sulph is for fluid engorgement problems or humidity. Swellings. Fluids. Lunar changes. A transit of the Moon wouldn't last that long, but a lunar progression could. It's an excess water eliminator. So if you are having fluid problems in the body, Nat Sulp is the cell salt to take. If you notice that damp weather bothers you, try Nat Sulp. I find that a lot of people are affected by the weather.

KALI MURIATICUM – GEMINI

The next one is the Gemini cell salt Kali Muriaticum. This is called the children's remedy and deals with the health issues of children. Also, sluggish conditions in the body. Rheumatism. It is a blood conditioner. You take it with Ferrum Phos to relieve any kind of inflammation or irritation. Also for constipation. These are all helped by Kali Mur.

CALCIUM FLUORIDE – CANCER

Calcium Fluoride is good for the enamel of the teeth. It is an elastic tissue builder. It is good for muscular weakness. For cracks in the skin. Piles. All of these can be helped by Calc Flour. Cracked lips. Muscular conditions. Any loss of elasticity in your body can be helped by this cell salt.

MAGNESIUM PHOSPHATE – LEO

Magnesium Phosphate is Leo's cell salt. It is useful for anti-spasmodic conditions. Motor nerves. An anti-pain cell salt. A nerve stabilizer. It is useful for cramps, neuralgia and pains in your body.

Audience: What amount of cell salts do you take?

DC: As far as amounts go, if it's an acute condition you can take the cell salt up to ten times in a day and stop. Otherwise, some are taken four times a day until the condition is relieved. You have to study the books and figure out your condition. I tend to take two at a time. They are called pellets and melt under your tongue.

If I'm having some type of problem, I'll take two of them such as for dental conditions. The rule is that the pellet must go from the bottom of your hand onto your tongue or underneath your tongue. You shouldn't let the salts drop on anything. There is something very etheric about them. Why do they work? They've been pulverized down to minute amounts. It has something to do with electro-magnetic ions that have actually been measured.

Cell salts apparently go straight to the cells where they are needed. Unless it's really something severe, start with two pellets and then see how your feel.

KALI SULPHURICUM - VIRGO

The next cell salt is Kali Sulphuricum (Kali Sulph) which is the cell salt for Virgo. If you have Saturn in Aquarius or a problem with oxygenation, this cell salt could be useful. It works with Ferrum Phosphate as an oxygen carrier. Ferrum phosphate, which is the cell salt for Pisces, is supposed to be taken along with the other cell salts. It helps utilize iron in the body. Kali Sulph is good for skin eruptions; it's an oxygen exchanger. Also, Kali Sulph is useful for bronchial problems; also scaling on the skin.

NATRUM PHOSPHORICUM - LIBRA

The Libra cell salt is Natrum Phosphoricum. It is considered a flu remedy. It is useful for gout. It's an acid neutralizer in the body. Instead of taking a product like Tums for the tummy, you could try Nat Phos. Also take it for digestive upsets, heartburn, rheumatic pain. This would be a good test to try taking Nat Phos the next time you have heartburn instead of an over-the-counter remedy and see if it works for you.

CALCIUM SULPHATE – SCORPIO

Calcium Sulphate is effective for abscessed teeth, removing toxins in the body and minor skin ailments. It is considered to be a blood purifier.

SILICA – SAGITTARIUS

The next one is Silica which is the cell salt for Sagittarius. It aids brittle nails, bones and vision. It can help you with tiredness and exhaustion. It is good for the hair. So is an herb called Horsetail. It's a cleanser in the body. Good for boils, pus. Silica is considered the most dangerous of the cell salts as it has a cutting action like glass in the body. You should take it in moderation.

CALCIUM PHOSPHATE – CAPRICORN

The Capricorn cell salt is Calcium Phosphate. It is useful for rheumatism and arthritis. Also poor nutrition. It's a tonic for the body such as when you're getting a Neptune or Saturn transit. Those two planets call for tonics. It can give you some pep and vigor.

NATRIUM MURIATICUM – AQUARIUS

The next one is Natrium Muriaticum which is the cell salt for Aquarius. This aids hydration in the body. It puts the moisture back in your cells. It regulates the moisture between the cells. It also controls the amount of hydrochloric acid that enters the body during digestion. You need hydrochloric acid in your stomach to digest food. It even helps in cases of sunstroke. If you are out in the sun and become dehydrated, this is the cell salt to take along with drinking water. It's a water distributor in the body.

FERRUM PHOSPHORICUM – PISCES

Ferrum Phos is the cell salt for Pisces. It helps increase hemoglobin so it has to do with the iron content of the blood. It builds blood vessels. It's a healer – for a cough, cold or chill. Anything that ends in "itis" according to the medical astrologer Dr. William Davidson (deceased) is helped by Ferrum Phos.

Those are the 12 cell salts also known as tissue salts. I have food sources for them also which are given in *Astrology and Health*. If you are getting your nutrition from food and don't like taking supplements, try the food sources. The Jansky books listed below have a lot of information on the cells salts also.

Kali Phos: green vegetables, potatoes, onions, apples and walnuts
Nat Sulph: beet root, cauliflower, cabbage, spinach, cucumber and onion

Kali Mur: oranges, peaches, plums, pears, tomatoes and sweet corn

Calc Flour: egg yolks, rye flour, most proteins and vegetables

Mag Phos: whole wheat bread, barley and rye, apples, lettuce, cabbages, cucumbers, eggs, walnuts and fish

Kali Sulp: carrots and most salad vegetables, whole wheat, rye and oats

Nat Phos: watercress, carrots, spinach, peas, celery, beet root, apples, raisins, almonds, figs and leeks

Calc Sulph: onions, mustard, garlic, cauliflower, leeks, turnips, radishes, figs and prunes

Silica: fibrous matter of fruits, vegetables and cereal and the skins of fruits and vegetables which usually gets discarded

Calc Phos: spinach, cucumber, lettuce, figs, plums, strawberries, lentils, almonds, wheat, barley, rye, fish, milk

Nat Mur: spinach, lettuce, chestnuts, cucumbers, lentils, carrots, cabbage, apples, strawberries

Ferrum Phos: lettuce, radishes, spinach, strawberries, lentils, onions and barley, the water from cooked vegetables

In *Astrology and Health* Sheila Geddes says that the tissue salts are one form of medication that can be used safely by the layman. She states that any amount taken which is surplus to the requirements will be eliminated by the body with no harmful effects. They can be easily purchased in tablet or pellet form in any health food store or pharmacy which sells homeopathic remedies.

HERBS AND PREDICTIONS

Here are some herbs and foods that could be helpful during various planetary combinations of transits, progressions or directions. Just as a precaution, you should be careful with herbs as they can sometimes have a toxic effect, so you don't want to use them indiscriminately. They can be toxic if taken in high quantities. One herb that you should avoid in large quantities is Goldenseal. After three weeks, you should stop taking it. Goldenseal can be toxic.

There are Chinese herbalists who have potent combination for various health problems. Herbs are different than the homeopathic remedies as they can have possible side effects. The NCGR 1996 "Memberletter" has a section on using herbs for the 12 signs of the zodiac.

You may be getting a Moon Venus combination. For example the progressed Moon is aspecting your Venus in some way. You may experience water retention or a water imbalance in the body. Bilberry would be a useful herb to take. Now this also works in reverse such as a Venus direction to your Moon.

Let's say you are getting a combination of Mars Uranus or Venus Uranus which affects the nervous system. It could be in any combination. Jupiter Uranus, Mercury Uranus combinations also. Bergamot, skullcap and valerian are useful for nervous complaints. Also balm and borage. These are all teas to help you calm down and sleep better. Ginseng is a tonic for the nervous system. Hops – if you put it in a pillow or a drink is also for the nervous system.

You can have Neptune transits that make you anxious and nervous as you can be walking around confused or unsure. Neptune can create anxiety. So these same herbs can also be useful under Neptune. There are homeopathic remedies for anxiety that I mentioned earlier.

Let's say you are getting a Mars transit that can cause fever. Balm is an effective herb. By the way, I never predict health problems. I would not say to someone you are getting Uranus to Mercury so you will have a nervous breakdown. Rather I would describe it as a period of stress and let the client know the time span of the transit.

Catnip tea for energy and a fever. Also licorice. Licorice is considered a women's herb.

You know that ginger is used for nausea and seasickness.

You're getting a Pluto transit. You're going through a transformation. A Pluto transit can also be a need to detoxify. A nutritionist can help you with a detoxifying diet. You can have fresh lemon juice every morning. Squeeze a lemon in warm water and drink it. It helps to clear up mucous in the body. Also asparagus, figs and parsnips are good for a Pluto transit.

Mercury Saturn combinations could lead to respiratory disorders – black currants for throat infections, fenugreek in a tea, sage to gargle with and uva ursi for respiratory disorders. Uva ursi is also used for cystitis. Coltstfoot for hoarseness, coughs and colds. Anise, licorice, garlic, ginger and sunflower for bronchial troubles or coughs.

Moon Mars can indicate stomach disorders. Arrowroot, cloves, honeysuckle and fennel are useful.

Blood problems can show up with the following combinations: Moon Mars, Jupiter Saturn, Moon Jupiter, Mars Jupiter, Mars Saturn, Mars Neptune: Nettles checks the flow of blood. Borage is a blood purifier. Red clover is a blood purifier as well as is dandelion.

Hyssop regulates blood pressure. (Always see a doctor to have your blood pressure checked.)

Herbs can be taken in capsule form or made into a tea. Usually you have to sip the tea all day to have an effect. You pour boiling water over the herb and let it seep for a few hours to get the effect. After a day or two stop taking the herb and see if you notice an improvement.

Sometimes combination of Jupiter and Saturn can have to do with the liver and Venus Saturn combinations can have to do with the kidneys. So you can take parsley as a kidney tonic, dandelion for both liver and kidneys; it is a general tonic for both. Thyme and rosemary for the liver and agrimony to tone the liver. Bay dissolves obstructions in the liver and the spleen. Chicory for liver impurities. Feverfew strengthens and cleanses the kidneys. Feverfew is also supposed to help against headaches especially migraines. Horseradish – kidney trouble. And mustard packs for back pain – possibly a transit of Saturn to your fifth house could indicate back pain.

Audience: What would be effective for a Saturn Uranus combination?

That could be a remedy for tension. You need something that relieves tension and anxiety. You are trying to make structural changes with Saturn Uranus. You can try homeopathic remedies: Nux Vomica for irritability and impatience. And Tuberculum and Ignatia if you get tension or circulatory problems with a Saturn Uranus transit.

MORE PLANETARY COMBINATIONS AND REMEDIES

For Saturn Sun combinations – vitality problems and poor resistance, colds and chills. Also fear. Arsenican Album.

I would look up in my sources anything describing a cold but you need to know the particular symptoms of your cold.

Sneezing, Silica, Nat Mur.

So if you are getting a cold, it depends on your other symptoms as to what remedy to take.

Redness of your nose: Silica.

Loss of smell: Mag Phos

Audience: What about dry mouth?

Dryness of the lower lips, skin falls off in large flakes: Kali Phos

After eating fatty food: Pulsatilla

Salivary disorders: mouth dry, person restless and anxious: Arsenicum. To be taken every two hours up to ten doses.

Mouth dry and hot, person feverish: Belladona

Lips dry and parched, great thirst and fever: Byronia.

Mouth dry and burning: Capsicum,

Tongue sticks to roof of mouth: Nux mosch

I also wanted to mention that for anxiety I have been told that the Rescue remedy, one of the Bach Flower Remedies, is useful. So if you are getting Saturn Neptune or Moon Saturn, you might try that.

Muscle problems: Arnica.

Sleep problems in connection with a Uranus transit: Before midnight: Coffea. Waking up between midnight and 2 AM: Arsenicum

There are specific remedies for the exact hour you awaken or can't sleep which you can find listed in many homeopathic books.

Moon Saturn: mental and emotional pain: Ignatia.

Saturn Mercury: mental attitude problems: Kali Phos.

respiratory disorders: Nat Sulph. Nat Mur or Mag Phos for neuralgia problems or Hypericum for nervous injuries.

I was taking Hypericum once for tooth sensitivity to cold and found it helped.

Saturn Mars: muscle joint pain, bruising: Calc Flour or Ferrum Phos and Kali Mur taken together. Rhus Tox for sprains.

Spasms which could be Mars Uranus combinations: start with Arnica, then switch to Ruta.

Saturn Neptune: anxiety: Aconite and also Phosphorous.

Uranus transits in general: Mag Phos.

Mars Uranus combinations: insomnia: Arsenicum.

Some remedies are good for more than one ailment.

Audience: How would you describe a Sun Moon opposition?

It could be an eye problem; it can be vitality problems. You might want to take nutrients for vision or teas such as eyebright tea for the eyes. Sun Moon in hard aspect can also indicate fluid problems. Unless the Sun Moon aspect is tied in with outer planets, it shouldn't be a long-term problem. Sometimes it's emotional problems.

Nervous system: Nux Vomica and Kali Phos.

Mars Pluto, Saturn Pluto problems. Overexertion. Rhus Tox.

All inflammatory problems: Ferrum Phos.

Urinary problems, cystitis: Aconite. Calcea can also be used.

At the beginning of the chapter it was discussed how to determine what remedy to take. You just can't take a remedy arbitrarily. You have to consider the symptoms. Here is a good example for women who are having menopausal problems and who get hot flashes. Lachesis is one of the remedies recommended for hot flashes and another one is Pulsatella. Now here's the difference.

Lachesis is for hot flashes that are particularly difficult in the morning. Pulsatella is for hot flashes around the face. Then there's Ignatia. Hot flashes along with constipation. Belladonna: hot flashes and headaches. Sulphurica: use when hot flashes are extreme.

Again, you find the remedy that fits your symptoms. And you can experiment with a different remedy, cell salt or herb. Just be careful of self-diagnosing yourself. If you have a serious illness, you shouldn't be treating or diagnosing yourself. Obviously, you would see a doctor. You strain a muscle at a health club or you have a stomachache. I wouldn't call a doctor for those problems unless it's so severe you are immobilized. I think that with most minor problems, you can treat yourself.

Arnica is helpful for the following. Mars Saturn. Mars Uranus. Wounds, bruises, and falls.

Here's one for puncture wounds. Ledum. Mars. A Mars transit can cause puncture wounds.

Fever and inflammation. Sun Pluto. Sun Mars. Aconitun. And Ferrum Phos at the beginning.

With all these cures, it's study, experiment and using preventative measures. We saw that if you eat a wide variety of foods you will get the food sources for the cell salts as well as vitamins and minerals. There are a lot of supplements out there but you have to remember to take them every day and they can get expensive. I think if you are in good health you don't need too many. If you start getting run down, supplements such as blue green algae and multi-vitamins could be of benefit as well as cell salts. And what if you are having pain from using a computer mouse, for example. Or indigestion from overeating. Or mental exhaustion from working too hard. These are problems you should be able to treat with cell salts, homeopathic remedies or a herb.

SOURCES

Chapman, J.B., M.D. and Perry, Eduard L., M.D. *The Biochemic Handbook,* Formur Inc., St. Louis, Mo, 1976.

Cramer, Diane: *How To Give An Astrological Health Reading,* AFA, Tempe, AZ, 1996.

Geddes, Sheila: *Astrology and Health,* The Aquarian Press, Wellingborough, Northhamptonshire, 1984.

Jansky, Robert Carl: *Astrology Nutrition & Health,* Para Research, Rockport, Massachusetts, 1977.

Jansky, Robert Carl: *Introduction To Holistic Medical Astrology,* American Federation of Astrologers, Inc., Tempe, Arizona, 1983.

Jansky, Robert C.: *Modern Medical Astrology,* Astro-Analytics Publications, Van Nuys, California, 1978.

Lockie, Dr. Andrew, *The Family Guide to Homeopathy,* Simon & Schuster, New York, 1993.

Powell, Eric, F.W. *Biochemic Prescriber,* Health Science Press, Devon, England, 1976.

The Smart Guide to Homeopathy, Boiron USA, Newtown Square, PA. 1-800-264-7661.

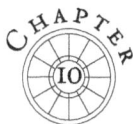

TOOLS IN MEDICAL ASTROLOGY

This chapter introduces the reader to three techniques that can give additional information in a health reading. You will learn how to read and understand a decumbiture chart (a chart for the moment of a diagnosis or the moment you take ill). You will see the effects of eclipses during times of illness. And you will learn how to read the South Nodal Chart, a chart that can be used along with the natal chart to point out weaknesses and sensitive points in the body.

This chapter includes techniques to help fine tune your medical astrology knowledge. They are in addition to the general steps in reading a chart in terms of medical astrology. (See *How to Give an Astrological Health Reading*¹). I will discuss three separate methods:

1. The Decumbiture Chart. It is a chart for when you get ill.

2. The use of eclipses regarding health.

3. The South Nodal Chart.

THE DECUMBITURE CHART

Though this may be new to some of you, it is a technique that goes back to William Lilly's time. And the chart has to do with the moment that you take ill.

It's the moment you lie down or as they used to say, when you take to your bed. Or it can be the moment a doctor says to you that you have such and such a disease. Or it's the moment you feel sick. And what if you can't remember any of those things. Well, then it could be the moment that you go to an astrologer and you could call it the moment of consultation because you may not always know the time you got sick.

Audience: The moment you lie down?

DC: Yes, The moment you lie down; the moment you don't feel well. During the Middle Ages it was the moment the physician looked at your urine. (The color of the patient's urine was used to determine the treatment.) That was the moment of the decumbiture. Now days, if you're not lying down, it's not that moment yet. It's that moment when you just can't get up. That's the moment of the decumbiture. Or you go to the doctor and he or she says that you have such and such a disease. That's the moment to be aware of and that's the chart I have here for the women with Parkinson's disease. It was the moment she and her husband remembered that the doctor said, "I believe you have Parkinson's disease." That's the time of the decumbiture. How many people really remember when they're told something? When I fractured my foot I didn't really remember exactly what time it was and when the doctor said it was a fracture, I don't even remember what time

268

that was. You think you're going to pay attention. You're supposed to remember because you're an astrologer, but I couldn't even remember myself. So it's not always the easiest thing to remember. So if you have no idea of when the illness began, but you call an astrologer and say you'd like a chart on your illness, the astrologer can do the decumbiture for the moment of the phone call. It's still valid.

Audience: What about your own chart?

DC: If you do your own chart, it's the moment you got ill.

Audience: Can you do it for the moment you make the chart? Like I want to make my chart now.

DC: Well, in your case that would be a horary chart. When the question becomes important you ask it. That's not a decumbiture. I would just say it's the moment you really feel ill. And we're not just talking about a 24-hour virus. We're talking about something more serious. According to Devores Encyclopedia of Astrology[2] it's called a lying down. So that's the meaning of a decumbiture. It's an event chart.

The Jane Ridder Patrick book on medical astrology has information on the decumbiture. (*Handbook of Medical Astrology* by Jane Ridder Patrick[3]) *Astrology and Health a beginners* guide by Dylan Warren Davis[4] has information on the decumbiture. I will give you enough information that you don't have to buy any books unless you want to. And then the original book, the bible of all these books, was Culpepper's *Astrological Judgment of Diseases* written in Middle English.[5] If you liked reading *Christian Astrology* by William Lilly, you'll enjoy this. Because most of the books you read now have already taken the Culpepper book and explained it in modern English. Later I'll quote from Culpepper, but it's that "what did he say?" type of English. And then you read it ten more times before you understand it.

Some astrologers read a decumbiture based on horary rules and do not use the modern planets. Jane Patrick Ridder does not use Uranus, Neptune or Pluto in reading the decumbiture. She will only read the chart if it's radical or if it's fit to be judged using the classical rules of horary astrology. Ridder would say that if the planetary ruler does not agree with the Ascendant, you are not to judge the chart. The same rule as horary astrology which says you can't read the chart if the Ascendant doesn't agree with the planetary ruler of the hour. I didn't get that feeling from the Thomas book, but he knows how to use all that ancient information on herbs. I look at the decumbiture as an event chart and read it based on the meaning of the houses and their rulers.

Refer to the natal chart of the woman diagnosed with Parkinson's disease. Symptoms include trembling and stiffness of muscles. It's a disorder of the nervous system, and it slows down your movement. Some of the most noticeable symptoms are trembling and sluggish movement along with stiffening. According to some medical astrologers, it's a Saturn Uranus problem; Gemini Sagittarius is also involved. She has a Saturn Uranus conjunction in Gemini. She even has Saturn parallel Uranus which intensifies the conjunction in longitude. She does have some of the significators of Parkinson's Disease. And the rigidity is shown by Saturn, the ancient ruler of Aquarius, her Sun sign.

PARKINSON'S
DISEASE

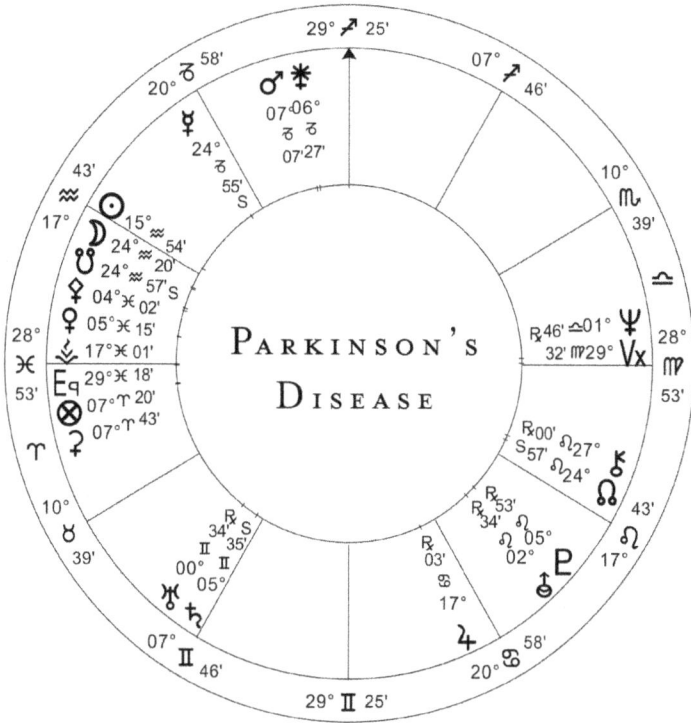

The nervous system is associated with Gemini. And her Saturn Uranus conjunction falls in Gemini. Aquarius can be involved with Parkinson's and she has the Sun in Aquarius and the Moon in Aquarius squaring Uranus, which could have to do with trembling and is another signature for Parkinson's. The muscle problem shows up as Mars Neptune. Mars is square Neptune and both fall in angular houses. Notice that Mars is also elevated in the chart. Also note the 29 degrees Gemini Sagittarius on the angles – critical degrees, the locomotive problems being Gemini Sagittarius, the 29 degrees meaning there could be something critical or a crisis in the life. And then you have Mars square an angular Neptune – muscle wasting. This shows up in the charts of people who can have a muscle problem. It can be a difficult combination. The muscles can become flaccid and weak. Neptune weakens Mars, which rules muscles. That's how you interpret it. In some charts Mars Neptune could be a lowered immune function. She also has a Jupiter Uranus semisquare – a spastic condition involving the involuntary muscles. And Neptune is square the Sagittarius MC which indicates a

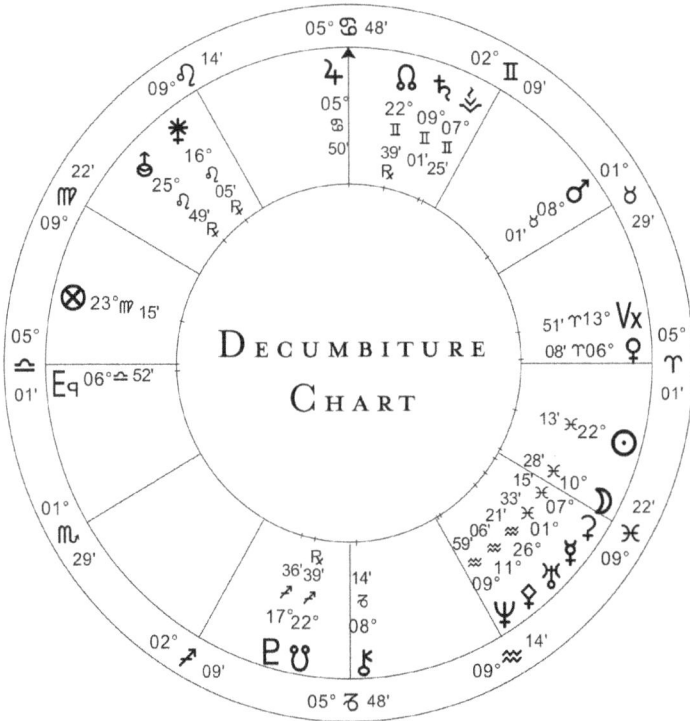

DECUMBITURE CHART

weakness in locomotion. Sagittarius can be a sign of loco-motion. Mercury is trine Uranus which could be a helpful aspect, but it's weak in that it's out of sign.

Mars is quincunx Saturn, which can be bone ailments and stiffness. Jupiter Uranus and Saturn Uranus are both spasm conditions. And also note that Mars is the focal planet in a Yod involving Saturn Uranus sextile Pluto. The Yod brings an element of fate into the chart. But probably the most difficult aspect is a hard aspect between Mars and Neptune involving angular houses.

Audience: Angular and hard?

DC: Yes, angular and hard is the most difficult. The planets would be angular and should be in hard aspect, or there can be afflictions involving the rulers of the angles. Remember the discussion of a mundane square in Chapter Two? This was the individual who had Lou Gehrig's disease. Mars conjunct the MC and Neptune conjunct the Ascendant. There's no aspect in longitude but they are in mundane square or in mundo. It's like having a Mars Neptune square in longitude. And that's a muscle wasting disease – Lou Gehrig's disease.

There's a lot more if we include midpoints, but I want to discuss how to read the decumbiture chart.

THE HOUSES IN THE DECUMBITURE CHART

The first house is the body, the health and the vitality of the patient. Therefore, with Libra rising Venus would be the ruler of the chart. The condition of the Ascendant and the condition of the ruler describes how serious the disease is. And you can see that Venus in Aries is deposited by Mars, which rules muscles.

The sixth house is the disease itself. The fourth house is the end of the illness or how long the illness will last.

Audience: Are all the houses used?

DC: No, they're not all used. I did skip around a little. The only houses that are used are the first, the sixth, the fourth, the seventh, the eighth and the tenth. And I came up with more information beyond the ancient rules so I could give you additional information.

The seventh house is the judgment or the physician or the astrologer. And the eighth house is the patient's death or surgery.

Audience: So if the seventh house is negatively aspected.

DC: It could be that you're getting the wrong information or advice from whoever is treating you.

The tenth house is the treatment, the medicines that are needed to help the patient. And I'm going to give you information on treatment that you can use for regular medical astrology too. You don't have to just use the information for the decumbiture.

PLANETS IN THE DECUMBITURE CHART

Now, the course and the enfoldment of the disease are described by the Moon. So we watch the progress of the Moon. Now, some astrologers will say to just look at the sixth house. Some say to just look at the Ascendant. You really have to look at all the relevant houses, and you have to see how the planets are aspected. But, in general, if the Sun is prominent, it's a short disease. A prominent Moon can indicate a recurring disease.

Audience: Chronic?

DC: Chronic would be Saturn. Recurrent means it comes and it goes. Literally. Mercury means it's changeable. Venus is neither long nor short, but it's not violent. It's sort of in between. Mars can be short and violent. And Jupiter is short. And Saturn is chronic. The ancients did not use the so-called modern planets – Uranus, Neptune and Pluto.

THE ASCENDANT IN THE DECUMBITURE CHART

So the first thing you look at is the Ascendant to see the vitality of the patient. If the Ascendant is in fire, the vitality is strong and there will be a quick recovery. If the Ascendant is in earth, it means that there is a sluggish metabolism and you may not be that robust. If it's in water, there can be weak vitality, or it can be an emotionally caused problem. You supposedly caused it yourself.

Audience: Could it be psychosomatic?

DC: Yes, it could be psychosomatic. Mutability is also psychosomatic. Water is emotionally based. Mutability is even more psychosomatic than water.

Air problems (this chart has air rising) could be caused by mental or nervous disorders. It means you're prone to a problem, but there's a certain amount of strength. In general fire is the strongest, air is next and earth and water are more or less equal in strength.

Audience: Earth and water are the same?

DC: Well, they're different in terms of the element but the same in terms of describing the vitality of the patient. As far as the elements themselves, there can be sluggishness with earth, but a lack of water can indicate too many toxins in the body. Excess water also has to do with the emotions as well as water-logged tissues. You also need to look at the natal chart. You have to take both the natal chart and the decumbiture into consideration. You would go back to the natal chart to see if there is too much or a lack of an element as was described in Chapter Five: "Rebalancing with the Elements and Modes."

Now we look at the Ascendant and see that it's in air so though she is vulnerable to illness, she has a certain amount of vitality. Maybe there's a nervous or mental component to the problem. A nervous component would make sense as it's Parkinson's and there's trembling. Then you take the planet ruling the Ascendant which in this case is Venus. Is it dignified or is weak? Look at the condition of the ruler of the Ascendant. In this case it's not dignified as Venus rules Libra and it's in the opposite sign; it's in Aries. However, it gets some fairly good aspects.

Now the ruler of the chart is weak because it's in detriment. If the ruler of the chart makes a hard aspect to Mars or Saturn, that makes the condition even worse. In this case Venus is in good aspect to Saturn. However, in one book I was reading it didn't matter if it was a good aspect or a bad aspect. It just said if the ruler of the chart aspects Mars or Saturn it wasn't good. It didn't matter if it was a sextile or a trine.

THE MODES IN THE DECUMBITURE CHART

In terms of the modes, if you have cardinal signs emphasized supposedly the disease ends very quickly. We know Parkinson's Disease doesn't necessarily end quickly. Fixed means that it's prolonged. And mutable is variable in length. And mutable is also very changeable.

I would say to take the cardinal, fixed and mutable modes to use as a description of the sixth house cusp and with Pisces there, it's variable – coming and going. And I also look at the Moon. And the last aspect the Moon makes is a square to Pluto, which is not good either. It's a difficult transformation. You want to watch the Moon. I'm going to give you more information on the Moon. The mutability means her condition is going to fluctuate, probably some days will be worse than others. It's going to be an up and down situation.

CRITICAL DAYS IN THE DECUMBITURE CHART

This was a method used hundreds of years ago which you can still use today. If you are experiencing an acute disease, you watch the aspects the Moon is making to see when the disease will flare up again. The Moon is used for acute disease. The movement of the Sun is used for chronic disease. You look at when the Moon is 45°, 90°, 135° and 180° away from its position in the decumbiture for critical periods. So you're looking at its aspects. I'll repeat that. When the Moon is 45° in aspect from itself, 90°, 135° and 180°; those are considered critical periods. However, if you're dealing with a crisis situation, then every time the Moon moves 22½° degrees which is one half of a semisquare which is one half of a square, that is a critical point in the day. This can get very minute, but it is a method of timing.

All these techniques in astrology can takes hours of investigation. These are the rules for the decumbiture chart. You have to watch the course of a disease yourself and see if it works that way. If it's a chronic disease, then you look at the Sun instead of the Moon. And when it's 45°, 90°, 135° and 180° further on from it's decumbiture position, those are considered to be critical days. You can basically watch what the Sun is doing to see how the disease is progressing.

Audience: You look at the Sun for chronic disease?

DC: Yes, even though Saturn is the planet ruling chronic disease. In the decumbiture the hard aspects of the transiting Sun to its position in the decumbiture are considered critical days. Also, you see when the Sun is aspecting difficult planets. Those could also be difficult days. When it's aspecting benign planets, the problem may ease up. And you can also look at the days the Moon transits the 6th house cusp, the 7th house cusp and the 8th house cusp for change. Basically, you can look at whatever you want if you like.

The critical periods are basically 45°, 90°, 135° and 180° aspects of the transiting Moon to its position in the decumbiture. Or if it's a real crisis, start looking at the transiting Moon every time it makes a 22½° aspect to its position in the decumbiture. And probably when it gets to a good aspect, whatever it is will start to alleviate. Which brings me now to treatment.

Audience: So you look at every aspect from 29 Pisces?

DC: No, from the Moon's position in the decumbiture, 10 Pisces. It's the transiting Moon to itself and the transiting Sun to itself and you can also look at the Moon to other planets.

When you read Culpepper he says, "Chronic diseases follows the motion of the Sun and 'tis about 90 days before the first crises appears. For in that time the Sun comes to the proper quartile of the place he was in at the decumbiture…but when he comes to his sextile or trine aspect of the place he was at the decumbiture, some motion appears a man, if he have any guts in his brains, may judge of the crises to come. Your fastest way to judge the disease is by the aspects from the Moon to the planets. When the Moon meets with the immical or of Saturn or Mars, have a care of your patient. And if you know what hinders by the same reason you may know what helps."[6]

Supposedly, her condition is going to be acute and it's going to come and go because of the cardinal sign on the fourth house cusp and the mutable sign on the sixth and the mutable Moon. I just felt that some days she'd be feeling fine, and other days the symptoms would come back. It's mutable. You will not be in constant pain all the time. Sometimes better, sometimes worse. Mutability. A fluctuating course of illness.

TREATMENT

The 10th house of the decumbiture chart is supposed to be what helps you or describes treatment options. So I've combined my knowledge of traditional medical astrology and some information on the decumbiture to give you treatment information. Refer back to Chapter Seven: "Recognizing and Treating Workplace Stress" for more treatment options. In natal astrology I look for an elevated planet in a chart and use it as a guide for treatment. For example, what are you going to do if you have a strong Sun in your chart? You are going to look for an expert to help you out. You're not going to treat yourself. You're going to go to someone who really knows what they're doing or who is an expert in a particular field of medicine. This is also true if the Sun is strong in the decumbiture chart.

Now if Jupiter and Saturn are strong in your chart, you're going to stick with traditional methods of healing. You're not going to do something really radical. And I also have a feeling that if Jupiter is strong in the chart there is a need for a liver tune-up. So if you see a strong Jupiter or a Jupiter problem, you might want to take some herbs to detoxify your liver. And herbs would also be shown by a strong Venus. You can choose any planet in your chart that you consider strong to describe how you should treat yourself in general. This is not just the decumbiture.

The Moon is fluids.

Audience: Is Mars exercise?

DC: Mars could be exercise or it could mean surgery. Now obviously if Mars is strong in your chart, you're not going to have surgery every time you develop a health problem so you have to think about what else Mars rules. It rules muscles so you could build up your muscles. Blood. Red corpuscles – build up the blood. Once you know the meanings of all the planets, you will understand what you need. Mars could also mean acupuncture since Mars rules needles. It is exercise, cauterization, surgery, but anything quick. Mars is fast. Don't wait around. The sooner the better. Now, Mercury, for instance, needs to read more about the problem at hand. Get out those books and figure it out. Consider your options. That's Mercury. You can teach yourself.

I mentioned Venus rules herbs. I also think a Venus problem means there's something out of balance in your body. Maybe your acid/alkaline balance is off. Something isn't balanced. So it's important to regain your balance in some way. Venus is involved with nutrition so perhaps you are not eating a balanced diet. You might just need to make some lifestyle changes. And anything that makes you feel comfortable is a Venus treatment. Indulge yourself. Possibly you have been working too hard. And maybe you're done a decumbiture and Venus shows up in a strong position. You might just need to have some fun.

Jupiter and Saturn are going to go the traditional way. With Saturn you might be helped by a chiropractor, a dermatologist or an osteopath. With Uranus you're going to try something radical. You might try something that involves electricity. Or a high-tech treatment.

Audience: Magnets?

DC: Yes, that's possible. I don't know about using magnets. I've read pros and cons on the subject. If you're going to use them, see an expert.

Audience: Energy healing.

DC: Yes, energy healing for Uranus.

Neptune. Biofeedback is associated with Neptune. Meditation. Also dreams, visualization, fantasizing. Interpreting your dreams. Some astrologers consider acupuncture to be ruled by Neptune as well as Mars. It's probably a Mars Neptune combination. Both Uranus and Pluto involve radical or unusual treatments. A strong Pluto in my opinion needs something to detoxify the body, to regenerate the body. And Pluto has to do with enzymes so you probably need more live enzymes, more raw foods in the diet. And if you believe in past lives you can do past life regression if you have Pluto strong in your chart.

Audience: What about fasting?

DC: Fasting is Pluto because anything extreme involves Pluto. I would also think Saturn would show up as you are depriving yourself of food as well as being disciplined and limited.

Audience: What about a bowel problem.

DC: Sometimes it's Pluto. Sometimes it's Mars. Sometimes it's a Scorpio emphasis. It could also be an 8th house emphasis. The longer you study astrology the more you know there can be more than one way to show a particular emphasis or tendency in a chart. The significators will work, but they may show up in different combinations. For example, a Scorpionic problem may show up as a strong Pluto; it may show up as an eighth house stellium or it may show up with a Mars Pluto aspect. A bowel problem can even show up with a Virgo emphasis. And a Virgo Scorpio combination can also point to a bowel disorder. So you look for the significators and see if they are in the chart and the more significators there are for a specific health issue, the more the person can be prone to that disorder.

I've discussed how to look for the critical days and what

each house means. The decumbiture is an event chart. It's the moment when the doctor says this is what you have or when you take to your bed, that moment you get the flu and you know you cannot get out of bed. Look at your watch. That would be an easy way to learn the decumbiture. How long am I going to be sick with the flu? And if it's acute you could look at the Moon and say, "Oh, I feel better. The Moon just got to my Venus. Or I can't move. The Moon just transited my Saturn." And then you've got the different methods of treatment.

The Seventh House. If you have Saturn in the seventh house, the horary rule would say don't trust the practitioner, don't trust the astrologer. So be careful of taking advice from someone when you have Saturn in the seventh of the decumbiture, because they may not be giving you the right information. And I would probably say that with Neptune also. That's there's a problem with the diagnosis.

Audience: Do you put the natal planets in a bi-wheel?

DC: No, the decumbiture and also the horary are standalone charts. Bi wheels are done with your transits and progressions and with solar returns and so on. These charts are read by following strict rules. You will also look at the natal chart for information obviously, which is what we did. And if there's a good relationship between the ruler of the sixth house and the ruler of the Ascendant in the decumbiture, then there can be improvement. If there's a hard aspect between the ruler of the sixth house and the ruler of the Ascendant then there could be a worsening of the illness. And one source mentioned the 12th house, self-induced illness. If there's a strong emphasis in the 12th house, then potentially you caused your own illness.

Now, as mentioned, the 10th house is the medicine, the treatment that you need.

In this chapter I'm giving you three different techniques to think about when you're doing medical astrology. You still need to learn the basics of medical astrology.

Audience: Can we read your books?

DC: Yes, I read all the books I could find on medical astrology before I wrote my first book and I put it all together and wrote *How to Give an Astrological Health Reading (AFA)*. And I have significators of diseases in the book. You can also use my *Dictionary of Medical Astrology (AFA)* for significators and *Manging Your Health and Wellness* (Llwellyn) as a textbook on medical astrology.

ECLIPSES

Another useful tool is the use of eclipses. We will look at what happens when there are several eclipses around the time a person becomes ill. Now, this sounds out of left field. How did we get into eclipses? I just wanted to give you another technique and show how important it is to look at eclipses when people get ill.

Look at the chart that says Breast Cancer (2). This is a case that continued to worsen. We all get eclipses hitting points in our charts. An eclipse affects your health more if it closely aspects a personal point. If the eclipses just falls somewhere in a house without involving a planet, it doesn't have as strong an impact as when it hits a planet. So in the first chart there was a lunar eclipse on January 9, 2001 in 19 Cancer 39. Notice it opposes everything around her

BREAST CANCER
(2)

Ascendant which is the physical body and the 12th house which can be a house of confinement. She was diagnosed on January 1, 2001. So we have an eclipse opposite an entire stellium. Then there was a solar eclipse on June 21, 2001 conjunct Mars in 00 Cancer in the sixth house. Another eclipse occurred on July 5, 2001 in 13 Capricorn conjunct Jupiter in the 12th house. A solar eclipse on December 14, 2001 in 22 Sagittarius was widely conjunct the 12th house cusp. So now we've got another eclipse involving the 12th house. Then a lunar eclipse conjunct Mars, 8 Cancer 48 on December 28, 2001. Then a lunar eclipse in 5 Sag 04, May

26, 2002 conjunct the Moon, and on June 22, 2002 a lunar eclipse at 3 Capricorn opposite Mars, and then December 4, 2002, a solar eclipse in 11 Sagittarius on the Moon. This is a person who has gotten worse and worse. Eclipses are energizers; they energize the area they fall in.

Now look back at Carl Sagan's chart which can be found in Chapter Five, "Rebalancing with the Elements and the Modes." Now, I'm not teaching you eclipses. I'm just pointing out that the more eclipses there are, the more problems there seem to be especially if you're getting a lot of eclipses on personal points in your chart. And the pervious example was getting one eclipse after another.

Audience: Does the problem end when the eclipses stop hitting the personal points?

DC: Unfortunately, after they stopped hitting the personal points she had some difficult transits happening. And this was a case when I was told not to talk about the future. So I didn't. All I discussed was her natal chart. I was reading an astrology book about cancer and it said there's no oxygen in cancer cells and this chart has a lack of air. So I thought, of oxygen therapy. It doesn't work for everyone, but give it a try since cancer cells survive with no air. I was just trying to come up with information.

Carl Sagan died of bone marrow cancer on Dec 26, 1996. He also had a lot of planetary stations hitting points in his chart; so I would also look at the stations of planets.

When a planet is about to change direction; it's slows down and seems to stop moving. When it is going retrograde that's a retrograde station. You notice the little "R" in the ephemeris. That's the station. And when it goes direct, the day you see that "D", that's the direct station. Those are potent if they fall on something in your chart. So in Carl Sagan's chart there was a Pluto station in 28 Scorpio on March 1, 1994 opposite his Ascendant. He became ill in 1994. And then there was a Uranus station on April 30, 1994 opposite his Pluto. There was a solar eclipse on May 10, 1994 in 19 Taurus. His Sun is 16 Scorpio. There were other things, but I'm just picking out the stations and eclipses. So the solar eclipse opposed his Sun. Saturn retrograded in 12 Pisces on June 22, 1994 opposite his Mars Neptune conjunction. Mars Neptune is always a point of toxicity. Then Pluto opposed his Ascendant in 25 Taurus. And Pluto of course was going retrograde and direct. A solar eclipse occurred on Nov 3, 1994 in 10 Scorpio. Back to the Sun which is in 16 Scorpio and Venus at 14 Scorpio. And a lunar eclipse in 25 Taurus 42 fell on is his Ascendant, which is also the fixed star Algol.. And that's considered a very difficult rising sign as it's on a malefic fixed star. Now, again, I did not do the whole chart. I'm only pointing out to you how important it is to look at eclipses.

Now, we'll finish discussing eclipses with Robert Urich's chart. You can find his chart in Chapter One, "Planets in Medical Astrology" where he was first discussed. When he first became ill with cancer I remember giving a lecture and saying he'll get through this; he had Jupiter on his Vertex during the operation so the surgery appeared to be successful. Then the cancer recurred. And there was a lunar eclipse when he first got ill on April 4, 1996 in 14 Libra, which is on his Neptune in 10 Libra. It doesn't appear to be a major eclipse for him. And I remember when I was first examining his chart, I didn't see anything that alarmed me. There was a lunar eclipse in 4 Aries on Sep 26, 1996 square his Mars. Later there was a recurrence

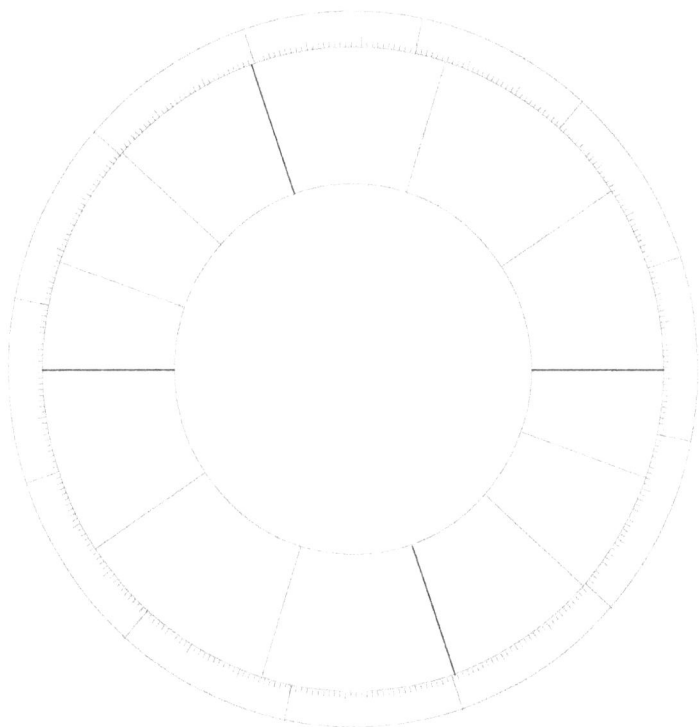

of the cancer. On July 5, 2001 there was a lunar eclipse at 13 Capricorn 39 square that same Neptune which was eclipsed when he first became ill. And on Dec 30, 2001 a lunar eclipse in 8 Cancer 47 also squared natal Neptune. Now Neptune does rule the immune system. And there was a solar eclipse at 22 Sagittarius 56 on December 14 2001 conjunct his Sun and opposite his Uranus. Notice his Uranus is 19 Gemini 26. His Sun rules his Ascendant so both indicators of the body were involved in that eclipse.

His Mars was eclipsed again on June 21, 2001 with a solar eclipse of 00 Capricorn 10. And he died in April 2002.

Audience: When someone is ill and then gets better, and then you see all these difficult eclipses what do you do?

DC: If they want to know, you tell them. If they don't want to know, and I have clients who don't want to know, you just do the natal chart to point out their weaknesses and what they could be building up in their body to help themselves. That's what I did with the woman with breast cancer who had all those eclipses affecting her chart. I did not say one word about the future because she didn't want to know. All I did was discuss the weaknesses shown in the natal chart that she could work on. And I talked about vitamins and minerals in regard to her chart. And I left it at that. You have to find out if people really want to know. They may not want to know. Do you want to know? As astrologers, we can't help but know where the planets are. You could just use the words "crises period." I always try to find a period of time that I can say looks good even if it's not for a few years. I still look for a date down the road. And sometimes they will make it that far and sometimes they won't.

Audience: Could you have used a decumbiture chart? Would you use a new one when Robert Urich got sick again?

DC: I would use the first decumbiture chart. I would probably set up a new one also when the illness returned.

THE SOUTH NODAL CHART

I want to introduce you to the South Nodal chart. There is a blank chart included on page 288 so you will be able to create your own South Nodal chart.

This is a chart that Robert Cark Jansky learned about in England. It's written about in two of his books: *Introduction to Holistic Medical Astrology*[7] and *Astrology, Nutrition and Health*.[8] I'm going to give you two samples of the South Nodal chart in action. The South Nodal chart is useful for finding weak points in your body. Robert Carl Jansky met a homeopathic physician in London who told him about the South Nodal Chart. You can use the blank chart form and put in your own planets in terms of the South Nodal chart.

In the South Nodal chart the Ascendant is considered to be the top of your body or your head and the Descendant would be your feet. It's a different way of looking at a chart. Just picture the body lying across the chart with the head at the Ascendant and the feet at the Descendant. The left side of the body are houses seven through twelve and the right side of the body are houses one through six. And you look to see where the planets fall in relation to the body. We'll use two examples and see how the chart worked out in Madeline Kahn's and Stephen Spielberg's charts. Then you can put in your own chart. (Madeline Kahn's natal chart can be found in Chapter Five, "Rebalancing with the Elements and the Modes.") Her South Nodal chart follows.

The cusp of the first house is your own natal South Node and Jansky says to use the True Node which in Madeline Kahn's chat is 3 Virgo 45. So what's the first house – 3 Pisces 45 which is her true South Node. And notice it's equal houses right after that. It's very easy. 3 Aries for the

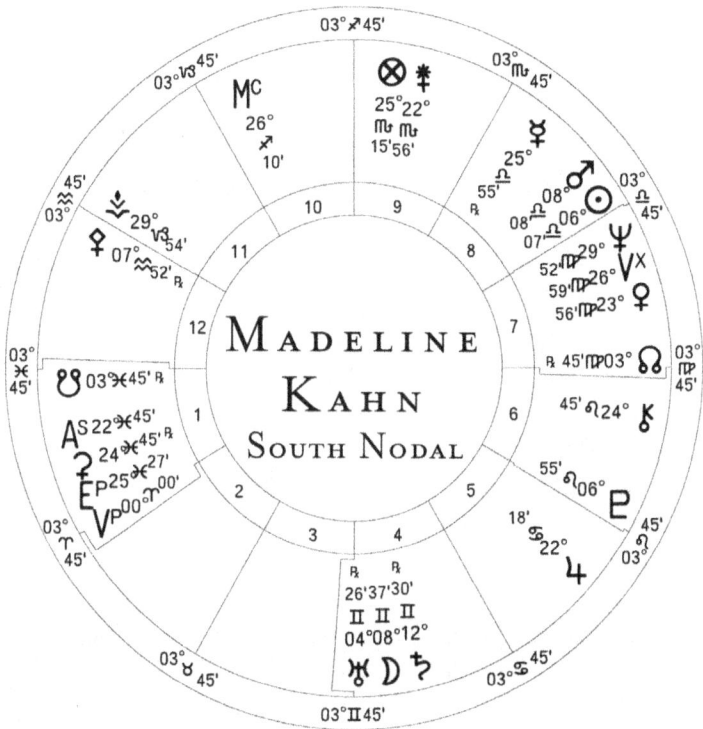

second house, 3 Taurus for the third house, 3 Gemini for the fourth house, 3 Cancer for the fifth house, 3 Leo for the sixth house, etc. You can add the minutes also. So, put your own South Node on the first house cusp and then equal houses around the wheel.

Audience: My South Node is around 8 Capricorn.

DC: Then you would put 8 Capricorn at the Ascendant and then put 8 Aquarius as the second house, 8 Pisces as the third house, etc. and go all the way around using equal houses. Label the inside of the chart South Nodal chart so you'll know what it is when you look at it in the future.

Audience: Do you put the planets in?

DC: You can put the planets in after you label the house cusps. You have to put the planets in to see how the chart works. In terms of computer programs, the Janus program has an option to create a chart starting with the South Node at the Ascendant. Otherwise you have to use blank chart paper and insert the houses and planets manually.

In the South Nodal chart you're seeing the head at the top or at the Ascendant and the feet at the bottom or what is normally called the Descendant. Number the houses beginning at the Ascendant. Houses 12 and 1 indicate the head area. Those are your feet opposite the Ascendant. The closer to the Ascendant a planet falls, the closer it falls anatomically to the top of the head. The closer a planet is to the second house cusp the closer it is anatomically to your neck or your collarbone. Remember, the position of the planets can indicate an influence in that part of the body in terms of the South Nodal Chat. The 12th and 1st houses are the head and neck to the collarbone. Then you read houses 2 and 11. Because you're dealing with the left and right sides of the body, you're combining houses. So 12 and 1 together make the head. House 12 is the left side of the head; house 1 is the right side of the head. You won't know if this works in your own life until you study it.

You can probably find Robert Jansky's books on the Internet even though some of them are out of print. *Introduction to Holistic Medical Astrology* is out of print but *Astrology Nutrition & Health* is still available. I've had a lot of success in finding out-of-print books on the Internet. Jansky died of a heart attack.

The 2nd and 11th houses – the chest cavity from the collar bone to the diaphragm. And that includes the heart.

Audience: Is that 11 and 12 and 12 and 1:

DC: No, let's repeat that. It's 12 and 1, 2 and 11 and now we'll do 3 and 10 which includes the stomach, upper small intestines, liver, spleen, and the pancreas. Again, the left side of the body are houses 7 through 12, the right side of the body are houses 1 through 6. The influence depends on where the planets fall in the chart. Jansky said the South Nodal Chat didn't show everything, but he gave an example where he couldn't see a problem in the natal chart but when he did the South Nodal chart he saw the problem.

Houses 4 and 9: lower abdomen, rectum, kidneys, bladder, large intestine, reproductive organs.

Houses 5 and 8: upper legs, kneecaps, buttocks.

Houses 6 and 7: lower legs and feet.

Audience: Where is the spine?

DC: Well, I always learned that the upper spine was Leo and the lower spine was Libra in a natal chart. However in the South Nodal Chart it's the center of the chart – the line dividing the body left and right. You can literally draw a line down the center of the chart from head to toes.

Audience: What about the teeth?

DC: They would be found in houses 1 and 12 since the teeth are located in your head. We are not doing regular medical astrology where we take each sign and each mode and examine every little thing in the body. We're doing something called the South Nodal Chart, which is another way of looking at the body. So don't confuse one with the other. You can still use your other rules in looking at the natal chart. Using this doesn't prohibit that. This is in addition to the regular chart, or you might say it's another way of looking at your body.

Audience: Does this chart have to do with the natural rulers of the chart?

DC: It has to do with the figure of a body laying down with the head at the Ascendant and the feet at the Descendant. The rest of the body fits into the various houses in the chart.

Let's look at Madeline Kahn's chart. Madeline Kahn died of ovarian cancer. Refer back to her natal chart in Chapter Five with 27 Pisces rising. You see a Moon Saturn conjunction in the third house of the natal chart with Uranus conjunct the third house cusp and the Moon. Obviously, the Moon can rule the ovaries as it rules the sign Cancer which rules containers in the body. The Moon is afflicted which afflicts the sign of Cancer. Since the planets rule physiology and the signs are the anatomical locations in the body, Cancer rules the ovaries, but the action is ruled by the Moon. So the Moon, which rules the sign of the ruler of the ovaries is afflicted by Saturn and Uranus even though it's a Gemini Moon. In medical astrology, when a planet is afflicted it also afflicts the sign the planet rules.

Now when you look at Madeline Kahn's South Nodal Chart those three planets – Moon, Saturn and Uranus – move into the fourth house. And what's the fourth house of the South Nodal Chart – lower abdomen, rectum, kidneys, bladder, large intestines, reproductive organs and hips. So I felt that you could see stress in the part of her body that eventually became diseased when looking at her South Nodal chart. The ovaries would be part of the reproductive area of the body. It was not a third house problem that happened to her; it was a fourth house problem according to the South Nodal Chart. Don't try to relate the houses of the South Nodal chart to the houses in the natal chart. Again, Jansky said the South Nodal chart will not show every health issue and that everything you see will not necessary occur. It might point to other problems that you are not aware of or that are not that obvious in the natal chart.

Now Stephen Spielberg had a kidney removed early in 2000. I found some information in "Entertainment Weekly" magazine. He had a kidney removed in January 2000. An irregularity was discovered. Spielberg didn't divulge the exact nature of the problem. According to medical experts, a kidney can be removed for malignant growth, non-malignant growth and infection. Stephen Spielberg's Mars/Neptune midpoint equals Venus. And when you look in the *Combination of Stellar Influences,* it states danger of infection, disease of the kidneys and to me that sounded like a kidney infection.

Audience: What is Mars Neptune?

DC: The Mars/Neptune midpoint is the point of infection or toxicity in your chart. And Venus which rules Libra and in turn the kidneys falls at that midpoint in his chart. That description is in Ebertin[9] – kidney infection. When something is removed from your body or there's an amputation it's ruled by Pluto. Look at his South Nodal chart and look at Pluto in the ninth house of the South Nodal chart. And look back at your notes – houses 4 and 9: Lower abdomen, rectum, kidneys, bladder, large intestines, reproductive organs and hips. So we see the kidneys.

Audience: Did they say which kidney it was?

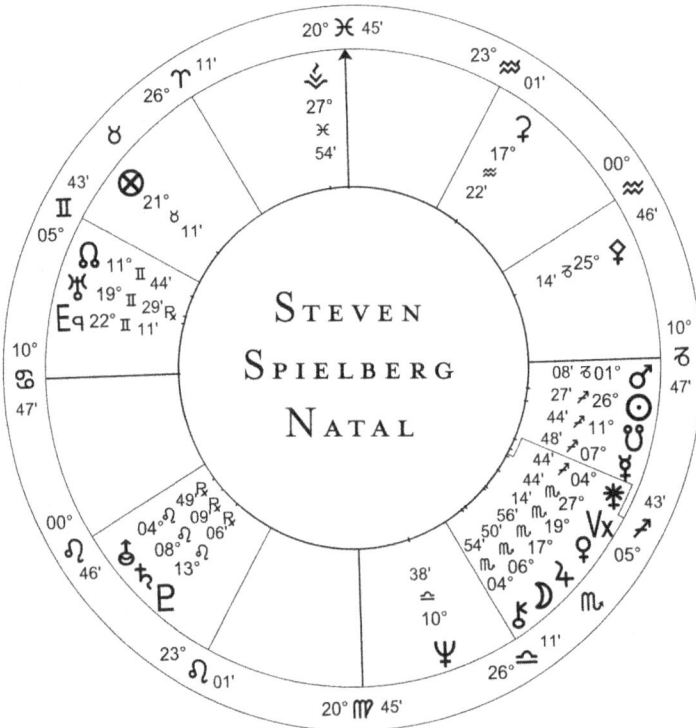

STEVEN
SPIELBERG
NATAL

DC: No, it wasn't mentioned. It would be great to know which one it was. I would just ask if the South Nodal chart shows anything? You can decide. Be aware that Pluto has to do with removals. And Pluto is also massive infection. Mars is infection. Pluto is a higher octave of Mars.

Audience: Does it have to do with Pluto in Leo?

DC: No, because too many people were born with Pluto in Leo. I'm only looking at the planets in the South nodal chart. I'm not looking at signs. Apparently you only look at the planets in the South Nodal Chart.

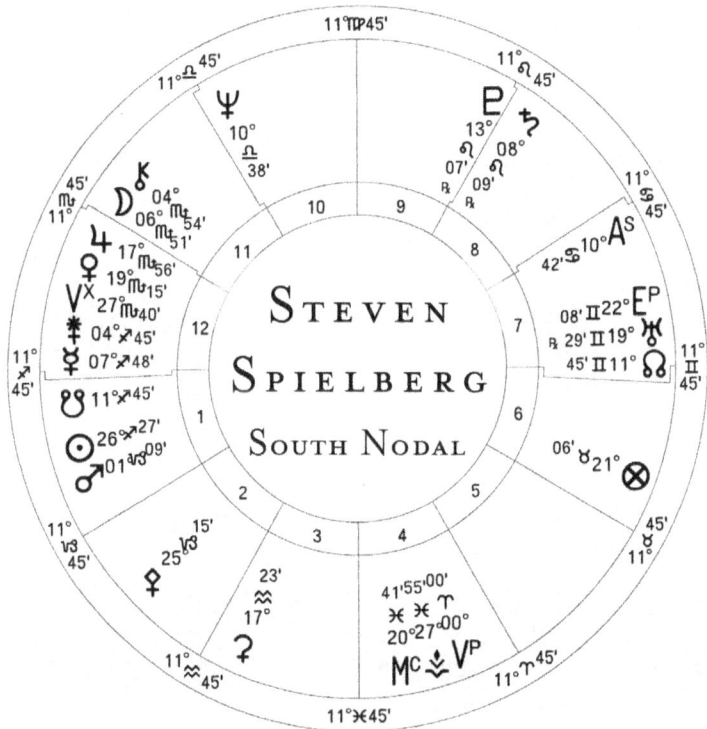

THE PLANETS IN THE SOUTH NODAL CHART

The planets have special meanings in the South Nodal chart.. You can look for where Mars and Pluto fall in the South Nodal chart for infection. And there can be surgery on the part of the body where Mars is or it's an area that can get very irritated. You can be injured where Mars falls in the South Nodal Chart. Scars are Mars. Look at your South Nodal chart and see where Mars falls and see if you have any scars in that part of your body.

You are very sensitive to touch where Venus is. You can be ticklish in that part of the body. This information is from Robert Jansky.

Audience: And Mars is surgery?

DC: Mars could be surgery but it is also where you can get inflamed, get an infection, have a scar, a bruise, a cut. Think of all the keywords for Mars.

Audience: And what about Pluto?

DC: Pluto can be a higher octave of Mars so it could indicate a more intense infection. It can also be a condition like parasites. It also rules removals.

Where Jupiter falls in your South Nodal Chart could be where you get fat. Or where fat accumulates. It's a larger part of the body. Check this out when you put your own planets into the South Nodal Chart.

Now Jansky said the location of the Moon is where you're sensitive to pain. I know one of the meanings of Mars is pain so Mars could be where you're injured and have pain and where the Moon is you're just very sensitive.

Body fluids may accumulate where the Moon is in the South Nodal chart.

Neptune – you are not in touch with that part of the body. Toxins may accumulate there. And possibly it's something hard to diagnose in that part of the body.

Uranus – nervous problems, tics, twitches, spasms. Jansky says that where Neptune or Pluto is there could be bacteria or viruses. Mercury would be nervous problems. Allergies – the Moon.

As mentioned previously, Saturn is underdeveloped, under active. Supposedly, the location of Saturn has the least blood supply. Therefore, it's the weakest part of the body. So you need to do something to build up that part of the body. Also, Neptune is a lack of tone. So basically look at the anatomical location of the signs that your Saturn and Neptune tenant. This is natal chart information. Build up or nourish those parts of the body as they are weak.

Audience: You said Saturn is under active and underdeveloped and the least what?

DC: It gets the least blood supply. Apparently, what keeps us healthy is blood going to a point or organ, and so where Saturn is located there isn't as rich a blood supply.

Audience: What if a planet is on the cusp?

DC: If a planet is on the cusp then, if it's in the first house, for example, but closer to the cusp of the second then it's lower down and closer to the collarbone. It depends on where the planet falls in relation to the location in the body. You may need an anatomy book to figure it out as far as the South Nodal Chart.

REFERENCES

1   Cramer, Diane L. M.S., *How to Give An Astrological Health Reading,* AFA, Tempe, AZ, 1988.

2   Devore, Nicholas, *Encyclopedia of Astrology,* Philosophical Library, New York, 1947.

3   Ridder-Patrick, Jane, *A Handbook of Medical Astrology,* Arkana, London, 1990.

4   Warren-Davis, Dylan, *Astrology and Health a beginner's guide,* Hodder & Slaughton, Headway, UK, 1998.

5   Culpepper, Nicholas, *Culpepper's Astrological Judgment of Diseases,* London, 1555.

6   Culpepper, Nicholas, pgs 14-15.

7   Jansky, Robert Carl: *Astrology Nutrition & Health,* Para Research, Rockport, Massachusetts, 1977.

8   Jansky, Robert. *Introduction to Holistic Medical Astrology,* AFA, Tempe, AZ, 1983.

9   Ebertin, Reinhold, *The Combination of Stellar Influences,* AFA, Tempe, AZ. 1972.

www.ingramcontent.com/pod-product-compliance
Lightning Source LLC
LaVergne TN
LVHW011217080426
835509LV00005B/178